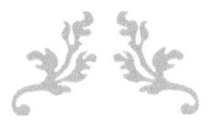

ESSENTIAL
NEUROLOGY

PROFESSOR ABDEL MAGID OSMAN BAKHEIT

MB (Hons), MD (Glasg), PhD (Glasg), MSc (Lond),
FRCP (Lond), Dip. Neurology (Lond).
Formerly Professor of Neurological Rehabilitation,
Universities of Plymouth and Exeter, UK.

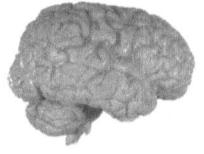

authorHOUSE®

AuthorHouse™ UK
1663 Liberty Drive
Bloomington, IN 47403 USA
www.authorhouse.co.uk
Phone: 0800.197.4150

Published by AuthorHouse 12/30/2016

ISBN: 978-1-5246-6770-2 (sc)
ISBN: 978-1-5246-6772-6 (hc)
ISBN: 978-1-5246-6771-9 (e)

Print information available on the last page.

Any people depicted in stock imagery provided by Thinkstock are models,
and such images are being used for illustrative purposes only.
Certain stock imagery © Thinkstock.

This book is printed on acid-free paper.

CONTENTS

CONTENTS

PREFACE

Neurological diseases are very common. They account for more than 10% of all diseases in Western European countries and North America[1], and result in 15 to 20% of all admissions to acute medical wards. Yet, only a minority of patients are seen by a neurologist during their hospitalisation. For example, one study has found that less than a third of patients with neurological disease who were admitted to the acute medical unit of a large teaching hospital in Britain had contact with the neurology services[2]. As most patients with neurological disorders are treated by non-specialists, a good working knowledge of the common neurological disorders is essential for medical students and all medical practitioners irrespective of their specialisation.

Most neurology textbooks are too detailed and also devote large sections to rare, obscure syndromes that have little relevance to practitioners outside the specialty of clinical neuroscience. The purpose of this book is to focus on the common neurological disorders that most doctors and other healthcare professionals are likely to see in their everyday clinical practice, and to provide up-to-date and concise information. The book consists of 15 chapters that cover, what I believe is, the essential knowledge required by a medical student, doctors in training, and by practitioners who are not specialists in neurology.

The approach that I have adopted in this book is to describe how the symptoms and signs are explained in terms of their anatomical location and their underlying pathology. Because a working knowledge of neuroanatomy is an important requisite for the accurate understanding and interpretation of most neurological signs, review of the regional anatomy precedes the description of the clinical syndromes where I considered this necessary. It is hoped this approach will facilitate a better understanding of the subject.

I deviated slightly from convention in arranging the chapters of this book. The text on management/treatment is usually the last chapter of textbooks. However, in a departure from this tradition, I have divided this section into two parts. This is because many neurological impairments, e.g. hemiplegia, dysphasia, apraxia, unilateral hemispatial neglect, etc., are present in most diseases of the nervous system irrespective of the underlying pathology. These symptoms require a management approach that is different from the medical treatment of the disease that caused them. To avoid repetition, I have summarised the management of the common neurological impairments in Chapter 2 to dovetail the description of the symptoms of these impairments and their clinical significance. The specific treatment of the various diseases, e.g. the antibacterial treatment of tuberculous meningitis or the use of anticonvulsants in epilepsy, is given in the relevant sections.

I hope that senior medical students, doctors in training and clinicians who are not specialists in neurology find this book a useful resource.

Professor A.M.O. Bakheit MB (Hons), MD, PhD, MSc, FRCP, Dip. Neurology
Birmingham, UK
April 2016

References
1. Neurological Disorders. Public Health Challenges. WHO, Geneva, 2006, ISBN 9241563362
2. Chapman et al. Acute neurological problems: frequency, consultation patterns, and use of a rapid access clinic. J R Coll Physicians Edinb 2009; 39: 296-300

CHAPTER 1

THE NEUROLOGICAL DIAGNOSIS

It is useful to think of the neurological diagnosis as a three-step process. The first step is to make a topographical diagnosis, i.e. to locate the lesion that is responsible for the patient's symptoms, because almost every neurological disorder has a tendency to occur in a specific part or parts of the nervous system. For example, the plaques of multiple sclerosis have a predilection for the visual pathways, cerebellum, brain stem and spinal cord. Therefore, localisation of a lesion to a specific part of the nervous system narrows down the number of possible diagnoses. However, since several diseases may affect the same part of the nervous system, the second step involves a further diagnostic workup to differentiate between the various possible disorders. The final step is to confirm the provisional clinical diagnosis with laboratory tests.

The topographical diagnosis is carried out by collating and analysing the patient's symptoms with the findings from the physical examination, and then assimilating these into a clinical syndrome. Special attention should be paid to the medical history.

1. General aspects of the medical history

As in other fields of medicine, the importance of a detailed and accurate neurological history cannot be emphasised enough. Apart from few specific points, the format of taking a neurological history is similar to that of general medicine. However, in contrast to general medicine, it is often necessary to ask neurological patients, at the end of the consultation, to repeat parts of the history because inconsistencies usually suggest impairment of memory or attention. Inconsistencies in reporting the symptoms are also an important feature of functional (conversion) disorders. It is also equally important to establish what the patient exactly means when he uses ambiguous words or phrases, e.g. collapsed, felt dizzy, etc. In addition, the clinician should allow the patient to describe his symptoms without unnecessary interruptions, and he should avoid asking leading questions. Enquiry should also be made about the onset, progression and course of the symptoms.

Some neurological symptoms may seem bewildering, bizarre or embarrassing to a layperson, and the patient might choose not to mention them for fear of ridicule. In other cases, cognitive impairment or a reduced level of consciousness may prevent the patients from describing their complaints fully or accurately. In these situations, information sensitively obtained from the patient's family members or an eyewitness is often invaluable.

2. The common symptoms of neurological diseases

Numerous symptoms result from neurological diseases, including headaches, convulsions, stupor, double vision (diplopia), slurred speech (dysarthria), difficulties with swallowing (dysphagia), focal muscle weakness, urinary and faecal incontinence, tremor, etc. More than one symptom is usually present. Assimilation of the symptoms with the findings of the neurological examination into a clinical syndrome enables the clinician to make a topographical diagnosis in most cases. However, sometimes patients present with functional symptoms (conversion disorder, hysteria) and it is important to recognise these symptoms in order to avoid unnecessary investigations and to prevent delay in the appropriate management of these patients.

Functional symptoms in neurology

Functional symptoms are complaints that cannot be attributed to clinically detectable structural and/or pathophysiological abnormalities of the nervous system or other organs. They can occur in children, as well as in adults. They affect both sexes, but are more common in females, especially those younger than 40 years old. Approximately two-thirds of patients presenting with functional symptoms have a psychiatric illness, usually depression or anxiety. Some patients with proven organic disease may also have functional symptoms. For example, an epileptic patient may present with genuine seizures and pseudoseizures.

Functional symptoms may mimic any neurological complaint, but by far the most common are pain, muscle weakness, non-painful sensory symptoms, dizziness, memory loss and pseudoseizures. Often the patient complains of more than one symptom. The onset may be sudden, insidious or episodic. Functional symptoms are often difficult to differentiate from malingering (i.e. feigned symptoms for personal gain) and also from hypochondriasis (health anxiety).

Features that help to distinguish functional symptoms from organic disease are clues in the medical history (history of mental illness, a recent significant adverse life event, frequent medical consultations, inconclusive laboratory investigations), the absence of hard physical signs of organic disease and the demonstration of inconsistency in the patient's clinical presentation. However, although inconsistency is one of the strongest indicators of the functional nature of a symptom, it should be emphasised that diurnal variability of genuine neurological symptoms and signs may occur. For example, the speech of patients with mild dysarthria may become unintelligible when they are tired, or an ambulatory patient with mild hemiparesis may start to drag his leg after walking a long distance.

3. The physical examination

The physical examination starts with an observation of the patient's demeanour and gait as he walks into the clinic. Some physical signs, e.g. tremor, are obvious even before any formal physical examination is carried out. In some cases, evidence of cognitive impairment, dysphasia, dysphonia or dysarthria is apparent from the patient's speech while he is reporting his symptoms.

A full neurological examination is time-consuming and may make the patient tired, or irritable and uncooperative. Therefore, the examination should be tailored to the condition of the individual patient and the clinical circumstances. However, in all cases a brief assessment of the patient's cognitive function and examination of the cranial nerves, motor and sensory systems is necessary. Sometimes valuable diagnostic information is often gained by repeating the neurological examination after a period of time.

The assessment of cognitive function

A few questions to assess the patient's memory, recall, orientation, mood and mental concentration are usually sufficient to confirm or rule out significant cognitive impairment. However, further screening tests, e.g. the Mini-Mental State Examination (MMSE) test, are necessary in borderline cases.

The methods of assessment for dysphasia, dyspraxia and hemispatial neglect are discussed in the next chapter.

The cranial nerves

A brief look at the patient's face is usually sufficient for the diagnosis of cranial nerve palsies. Ptosis (drooping of the eyelid), a convergent or divergent squint, and a dilated pupil are signs of lesions of the oculomotor nerves (III, IV, VI) and this can be confirmed by evidence of paralysis of voluntary eye movements. Facial asymmetry, a smoothed out nasolabial fold on one side, drooping of the corner of the mouth and the patient's inability to close his eye indicate a lower motor neuron facial weakness. A flaccid, large tongue with fasciculations (visible twitching of muscle fibres) is a sign of hypoglossal nerve palsy and a deviated, immobile soft palate suggests a lesion of the vagus nerve. However, although inspection often yields valuable diagnostic information, examination is necessary to detect lesions of the olfactory, optic, trigeminal, auditory and spinal accessory nerves.

The olfactory nerve – olfactory nerve function is tested by asking the patient to sniff different substances. Each nostril is tested separately. The test is seldom carried out in a routine clinical examination and usually has limited diagnostic value.

The optic nerve – examination of the optic nerve should include an assessment of the size of the pupils (normally the pupil is 3-5 mm in diameter in average light conditions), and the direct and consensual light reflex. (The direct light reflex is pupillary constriction in response to bright light, whereas the consensual light reflex is the simultaneous constriction of the other pupil.) In addition, the visual acuity, colour vision, visual fields and the optic fundus should be examined.

Visual acuity is usually measured with Snellen's chart and colour vision is often tested with Ishihara's pseudoisochromatic plates. (Ishihara's test plates consist of 38 sheets. Each sheet contains a circle filled with dots of different sizes and colours. A number, which is invisible to those with impaired colour vision, is embedded within the circle. The patient with reduced or absent colour vision is unable to read the number.)

The bedside assessment of the visual fields is made with the confrontation method. In this method, the examiner compares the patient's visual fields with his own fields. (The confrontation method assumes that the examiner's visual fields are normal.) Each eye is tested separately. The test is carried out with the patient sitting opposite to the examiner and continuously looking into one of the examiner's eyes while covering the other eye. The examiner moves an object (usually a hatpin) in front of the patient's eye and maps out the visual field by asking the patient to tell him as soon as he sees the object. The object is moved methodically from different directions in order to examine the whole visual field. The visual fields can also be measured with manual or computer controlled perimetry: a method in which the patient's visual field is plotted as a bright object is moved on a screen from the periphery into the visual field.

Examination of the optic fundus may reveal evidence of optic atrophy, papilloedema or other pathology. Optic atrophy is characterised by a very pale, small optic disc with well-defined margins. The retinal vessels usually appear normal. In the early stages of papilloedema, the margins of the optic disc are blurred, the physiological cup is full, and the retinal veins are engorged and non-pulsatile. Later, there are also extensive retinal haemorrhages.

The trigeminal nerve – the trigeminal nerve consists of motor fibres that innervate the muscles of mastication (the masseter, medial and lateral pterygoids and temporalis), and sensory fibres to the facial skin and part of the scalp. The sensory fibres divide into ophthalmic, maxillary and mandibular branches. The ophthalmic division supplies the forehead skin and the scalp, the mandibular division supplies the skin below the corner of the mouth, and the maxillary division supplies the remainder of the facial skin except the angle of the jaw. The ophthalmic branch also contains the afferent (sensory) fibres of the corneal reflex. (The motor fibres of the corneal reflex are part of the facial nerve.)

Examining the sensory division of the trigeminal nerve involves assessing the corneal reflex (a light touch of the cornea with a piece of cotton wool results in closure of the eyelids when the reflex is present), and the spinothalamic sensation in the trigeminal nerve dermatomes. The motor division is examined by asking the patient to open his jaw against the examiner's resistance and also to move his jaw laterally against resistance.

The auditory nerve – this nerve is tested by asking the patient to repeat words whispered by the examiner into the patient's ear, and also by performing Weber's and Rinne's tests. The Weber test is conducted by placing a vibrating tuning fork in the middle of the patient's forehead. The vibration is not heard or is weaker on the side of the lesion. Rinne's test is used to distinguish sensorineural deafness from conductive deafness. The vibrating tuning fork is placed on the mastoid process (to test bone conduction) and then held close to the ear (to test air conduction). Normally, air conduction is better than bone conduction. The reverse is true in cases of sensorineural deafness.

The spinal accessory nerve – the integrity of the spinal accessory nerve is evaluated by asking the patient to turn his head to one side and to shrug his shoulder against the examiner's resistance. This is to test the strength of the sternomastoid and trapezius muscles, respectively.

The motor system

Examination of the motor system is essential for the diagnosis of pyramidal tract lesions, extrapyramidal and cerebellar disease, and muscle disorders. The examiner should look for focal muscle wasting or hypertrophy, abnormal postures and movements (see Chapter 7), and also assess the muscle tone, muscle strength, coordination and tendon reflexes. Assessment of the patient's gait is also an integral part of the examination of the motor system.

The muscle tone is assessed by measuring the degree of resistance to the examiner's flexion and extension of the patient's limbs. The tone may be normal, reduced (hypotonia) or increased (hypertonia). There are two types of muscle hypertonia: spasticity and rigidity. In spasticity, there is initial resistance to the passive movement, which suddenly gives way as the movement is continued. By contrast, rigidity is characterised by waxing and waning of the resistance to passive muscle stretch; hence, it is often described as cogwheel rigidity.

In clinical practice, muscle strength is assessed by observing the posture and voluntary movements of the affected limb and by comparing the patient's muscle strength with that of the examiner. The scale of the Medical Research Council (MRC), which has the advantage of being simple and brief, may be used to record the degree of muscle weakness (see table 1.1).

Table 1.1
The MRC scale:

Grade	Description
0	No voluntary movement.
1	Flicker of a movement.
2	Movement is present, but only if the effect of gravity is removed.
3	Movement is present against gravity, but not against the examiner's resistance to the movement.
4	Movement is present against gravity and resistance, but weaker than the examiner's strength. (The comparison should make allowance for the patient's age and build.)
5	Full muscle strength.

The reflexes that are routinely tested are the biceps (C5), triceps (C7), supinator (C6), the knee (L4) and the ankle jerk (S1). In the absence of disease, the reflexes are symmetrical. Depressed or absent reflexes on one side are a sign of a lower motor neuron lesion. Brisk reflexes suggest an upper motor neuron lesion. Examination of the motor system should also include the Babinski reflex, which is a reliable sign of upper motor neuron lesions. (A positive Babinski reflex may be present in the absence of an upper motor neuron lesion in comatose patients, in the post-ictal phase of an epileptic seizure, and in infants.)

To elicit the Babinski reflex, the patient should be in the supine position with his leg fully exposed. The lateral border of the sole of the foot is scratched slowly with a blunt object, e.g. a key, starting on the lateral side of the heel and continuing upwards to the fat pad of the fifth metatarsal before turning medially towards the big toe. The strength with which the stimulus is applied should be proportional to what the patient is able to tolerate. In patients with very sensitive feet, a more meaningful response is usually obtained by stroking the lateral dorsum of the foot. Dorsiflexion of the big toe means a positive Babinski sign, i.e. an extensor plantar response. It is important to look for contraction of the proximal leg muscles (which may be subtle), as the flexor synergy of these muscles is an essential part of an extensor plantar response.

The equivalent to the Babinski reflex in the upper limbs is Hoffman's sign. The examiner flicks the patient's distal phalanx of the middle finger into flexion. A positive Hoffman's sign consists of flexion and adduction of the thumb and index finger.

Coordination in the upper limb is assessed with the finger–nose test. The patient is asked to touch, with his index finger, the tip of the examiner's finger and then touch his own nose. The examiner's finger should be positioned at an arm's length from the patient. A patient with cerebellar disease carries out the movement in a jerky and clumsy fashion (dyssynergia), and overshoots the target (dysmetria). There is also tremor as the patient's finger approaches the target (intention tremor). The equivalent test for coordination in the lower limb is the heel–shin test. In this test, the patient is asked to put his heel on the knee of the opposite leg and slide it down the shin. Dysdiadokokinesis is another sign of cerebellar disease. It is elicited by asking the patient to perform rapid alternating movements, e.g. quick pronation and supination of the forearm. Dysdiadokokinesis is the failure to execute the task smoothly.

Gait abnormalities are common in neurological patients and provide important diagnostic information as shown in table 1.2.

Table 1.2
The causes and description of the most common gait abnormalities:

Gait type	Description
Hemiplegic gait – upper motor neuron lesions	Circumduction with the paretic leg, the knee is extended throughout the gait cycle, the toes scrape the floor.
Diplegic (scissor) gait – bilateral upper motor neuron lesions	Stooped posture, the thighs are adduced, the knees are flexed and touching each other, the toes of both legs scrape the floor.
Ataxic gait – cerebellar or posterior column lesions	Broad-based, unsteady gait. The patient veers from the intended path and lurches from one side to the other.
Festinant gait – Parkinson's disease	Short, hurried steps, stooped posture, difficulties turning around, etc. See Chapter 7 for a detailed description.
High steppage gait – foot drop, sensory neuropathies	Excessive knee flexion during the swing phase of the gait cycle, inaccurate foot placement in stance.
Waddling gait – weakness of the pelvic girdle muscles	Broad-based and symmetrical. With each step, the pelvis drops on the side of the forward leg and rises in the stance phase of the gait cycle.

The sensory system

It is clinically useful to separate the sensory modalities into three groups: spinothalamic, posterior column and parietal lobe sensory modalities.

Spinothalamic sensation is the perception of light touch, pain and temperature. Light touch is tested with a piece of cotton wool applied to the skin and pain (pinprick) with a blunt needle. To test the temperature sensation, a cold and a warm object are used. In all cases, the testing should be carried out methodically in order to map out the distribution of the sensory impairment or loss, e.g. dermatome distribution, glove and stocking distribution, etc.

Posterior column sensation consists of joint position (proprioceptive) and vibration sense. To test the joint position sense in the upper limbs, the examiner randomly either flexes or extends the distal interphalangeal joint of the index finger and asks the patient to report the direction of the movement while his eyes are closed. To test the lower limbs the procedure is repeated by passively moving the terminal joint of the big toe.

Severe impairment of joint position sense in the lower limbs causes sensory ataxia only when the patient's eyes are closed because vision compensates for proprioceptive sensory loss. The ataxia is confirmed if the patient loses his balance when he stands up with his eyes shut. This is called Romberg's test.

Examination of the vibration sense in the upper and lower limbs is made with a vibrating tuning fork placed on the dorsum of the index finger or the big toe, respectively.

An important parietal lobe sensory function is the integration and interpretation of all sensory information that enables a person to distinguish objects by their form, size, shape and texture (stereognosis), and to accurately locate tactile stimuli (topognosis). It is not possible to assess the parietal lobe sensory function if the spinothalamic and posterior column sensation is absent or severly impaired. In order to test for stereognosis, the patient is asked to identify, with his eyes closed, an object (e.g. a coin) placed in his hand. Topognosis is assessed by touching part of the patient's body, also while his eyes are closed, and then asking him to locate the touch.

4. The main neurological syndromes

The localisation of lesions in the various parts of the nervous system and the description of the salient features of the main neurological syndromes are summarised in this section. Details of the methods of assessment and treatment of these syndromes are provided in Chapter 2.

4.1 The 'false localising' signs

Although most focal neurological signs indicate the site of the lesion that is responsible for their occurrence, some signs do not convey such valuable information. An example of these 'false localising' signs is sixth nerve palsy. It is often difficult to accurately identify the exact site of the lesion of this nerve because of its long course from the brain stem to the eyeball. Other symptoms and signs, such as headache and papilloedema, suggest raised intracranial pressure, hydrocephalus, or diffuse brain disease and do not indicate the site of the underlying lesion.

The syndrome of raised intracranial pressure

The syndrome of raised intracranial pressure (ICP) may result from brain disease as well as systemic disorders, and, as such, does not localise the lesion to any specific part of the nervous system. Large space-occupying lesions within the cranial cavity (such as brain tumours), massive cerebral oedema (e.g. due to severe traumatic brain injury) and obstruction of the CSF pathways are the most common causes. Other causes are chronic meningitis, cerebral venous sinus thrombosis, benign intracranial hypertension, hypertensive encephalopathy and chronic severe hypoxia.

The main symptoms of raised ICP are headache, nausea, vomiting, double vision and amaurosis fugax (blurring or loss of vision lasting a few seconds due to sudden increase in the already raised ICP, e.g. when coughing, sneezing or bending forward). The headache is typically worse in the morning and tends to improve as the day progresses. Abducens nerve palsy may be present. Examination of the optic fundus usually reveals evidence of bilateral papilloedema.

Hydrocephalus

The CSF is formed mainly by the choroid plexuses of the lateral ventricles and is absorbed by the arachnoid villi on the surface and base of the brain. An equilibrium between CSF formation and absorption maintains the circulating CSF volume at 150-170 ml. An increase in the CSF volume (hydrocephalus) results from a mismatch between production and absorption or from obstruction to the CSF pathways.

The most common cause of hydrocephalus is obstruction to the CSF flow from the lateral ventricles to the subarachnoid space due to brain tumours, subarachnoid haemorrhage, chronic meningitis or venous sinus thrombosis. Hydrocephalus due to excessive CSF production is rare. Its main causes are benign intracranial hypertension and papilloma of the choroid plexus. The cerebral CSF volume is also increased in patients with severe brain atrophy.

Hydrocephalus usually causes raised intracranial pressure (ICP). However, in some cases of chronic meningitis and subarachnoid haemorrhage the increase in the CSF volume is very gradual and does not raise the ICP. This condition is called normal pressure hydrocephalus. Its clinical presentation is different from that of obstructive hydrocephalus and consists of slowly progressive gait abnormalities, incontinence of urine and faeces, and cognitive impairment (Hakim's triad).

4.2 The cerebral cortex

Each region of the cerebral cortex acts as a separate functional unit and controls a specific function or functions, but this functional specialisation is not absolute. The different regions of the same hemisphere are interconnected by a network of white matter fibres known as the association fibres. These association areas are important for the integration of the sensory and motor stimuli within the same hemisphere. The connection between the two hemispheres is achieved through commissural fibres, namely the corpus callosum and the anterior commissure. Lesions of the different parts of the cerebral cortex and/or the association areas result in specific neurological syndromes.

The frontal lobes

The frontal lobe has three distinct functional areas: the motor cortex, the prefrontal cortex and, in the dominant hemisphere, Broca's area. (The dominant hemisphere is the hemisphere that contains the neurons responsible for language. It is the left hemisphere in most people.) The motor cortex lies immediately anterior to the central sulcus (the Rolandic fissure), whereas Broca's area occupies the inferior frontal gyrus of the dominant hemisphere. The remainder of the frontal lobe is referred to as the prefrontal cortex.

Unilateral lesions of the motor cortex cause hemiplegia on the side contralateral to the lesion. This is because, in the brain stem, the corticospinal tract fibres cross over to the opposite side. Parasagittal lesions cause paraplegia. (The motor nuclei for each leg are in the medial aspect of the frontal lobe.) Lesions in Broca's area result in expressive dysphasia. Bilateral damage to the prefrontal cortex results in cognitive impairment. Forced grasping, i.e. the involuntary (reflex) finger flexion and grasping when the palm of the hand is gently touched, arises from lesions of the supplementary motor area. Urinary incontinence, epileptic seizures and change in personality and behaviour are other features of frontal lobe lesions.

Broca's area and disorders of the language function
The neural structures that are responsible for language function are concentrated around the lateral sulcus (the Sylvian fissure). The neurons responsible for language expression and comprehension are located in the inferior frontal gyrus (Broca's area) and the middle and superior parts of the temporal lobe (Wernicke's area), respectively. Broca's and Wernicke's areas are connected by a bundle of fibres known as the arcuate fasciculus. Other language areas are the supramarginal and angular gyri of the parietal lobe and a network of deep white matter fibres. The language areas are in the left hemisphere in most people. Only approximately 10% of the world's population have their language function in the right hemisphere. Lesions of the language areas result in dysphasia. Verbal perseveration (unintended, continuous repetition of the same word or phrase) is usually associated with lesions of the head of the caudate nucleus. Mutism is due to fronto-putaminal lesions or large brain stem lesions.

The terms dysphasia and aphasia are usually used interchangeably to mean impairment of language comprehension, expression or both. The definition excludes the language and speech disorders that result from global intellectual impairment (severe learning disability or dementia), deafness or disorders of phonation. Language is the formulation and conveying of one's thoughts in words and sentences, and should be distinguished from speech. The latter is the articulation of language.

Both cerebral hemispheres are involved in language function. Instinctive language that conveys emotions and non-verbal communication, such as gestures and facial expression, is controlled by both cerebral hemispheres. By contrast, propositional language, i.e. the processes of inner thoughts and their external expression in spoken and written language, is associated with the left (dominant) hemisphere in right-handed people, and also in most ambidextrous and left-handed individuals.

Lesions of Broca's area cause expressive dysphasia. A detailed description and the assessment, differential diagnosis and treatment of dysphasia are discussed in Chapter 2.

Dysarthria
Dysarthria is a disorder of the articulation of speech. Dysarthric speech is slurred, slow and imprecise. It is often monotonous and lacks the usual variations in intonation and pauses, i.e. dysprosodic. Many non-neurological conditions, e.g. mouth ulcers, ill-fitting dentures, acute alcohol intoxication, may interfere with articulation and result in slurred speech. Numerous neurological disorders also cause dysarthria, including diseases of orofacial muscles, cranial nerves, brain stem, cerebellum and cerebral cortex.

The temporal lobe
The temporal lobe consists of three parts each of which has a separate function. These are the parahippocampal cortex, the hippocampus and the amygdala. The parahippocampal complex contains the primary auditory cortex. In addition, in the dominant hemisphere at the temporo-parietal junction, it contains the receptive language area (Wernicke's area). The medial part of the temporal lobe contains the hippocampus and the amygdala. These structures have an important role in the formation and

storage of memory and in the control of emotional responses, respectively. Part of the optic radiation also crosses the temporal lobe.

Sensory (receptive or Wernicke) dysphasia, temporal lobe epilepsy, cortical deafness (with bilateral lesions), auditory hallucinations, hallucinations of smell, disorders of memory and behaviour, and upper homonymous quadrantanopia are the main signs of temporal lobe disease. The most common pathological conditions of the temporal lobe are stroke, tumours, trauma and herpes simplex encephalitis.

The parietal lobe

The spinothalamic and posterior column sensory fibres converge in the thalamus where the initial processing the somatosensory information takes place. The information is then relayed to the parietal lobe. The main function of the parietal lobe is the integration of the somatosensory information with tactile, auditory and visual information in order to construct awareness of self, i.e. the relationship of the person's body parts to each other (the so-called body schema), and to the surrounding environment. The parietal lobe also plays an important role in visuospatial processing, discrimination of tactile stimuli and in the ability to manipulate objects. In addition, the parietal lobe contains some of the fibres of the optic radiation.

Lesions of the parietal lobe result in impairment or loss of the sensory modalities of stereognosis, topognosis and two-point discrimination on the side of the body contralateral to the lesion. In addition, lesions of the dominant parietal lobe cause ideomotor apraxia, and those of the non-dominant lobe cause left hemispatial neglect and constructional apraxia. Unilateral lesions of either parietal lobe also cause homonymous lower quadrantanopia. (For further details see the section on the visual pathways.)

Ideomotor apraxia

Ideomotor apraxia is a cognitive deficit characterised by the inability to carry out learnt, purposeful motor activities in the absence of significant upper limb muscle weakness, impairment of sensory function or poor comprehension of the required task. The condition is referred to as dyspraxia when the disability is partial. (However, as in the case of aphasia and dysphasia, the terms apraxia and dyspraxia are used interchangeably.) Ideomotor apraxia is seen predominantly after left parietal lobe lesions.

Ideomotor apraxia is broadly classified into limb apraxia and orobuccal (facial) apraxia. Sometimes the apraxic errors result from failure to follow the correct sequence of the different steps that are required to complete the motor task successfully. In these situations planning, rather than the actual execution of the motor act, is primarily affected and the patient is said to have ideational apraxia.

Limb apraxia should be distinguished from constructional and dressing apraxia. The latter disorders result from impairment of visual-spatial perception and are primarily associated with non-dominant parietal lobe lesions. Constructional apraxia is defined as the inability to assemble an object from its constituent parts. By contrast, dressing apraxia is characterised by difficulties aligning items of clothing to the appropriate part of the body. For example, a patient with dressing apraxia may insert his leg through a shirtsleeve while attempting to dress his upper body or may put on a garment back to front.

Unilateral hemispatial sensory neglect

Unilateral hemispatial sensory neglect is one of the most common and clinically important cognitive impairments in patients with neurological disease. It results from lesions of the inferior part of the non-dominant (usually the right) parietal lobe or the parieto-temporal junction.

Unilateral hemispatial sensory neglect (also called hemineglect, visual neglect or visual inattention) is a complex and multifaceted phenomenon that is characterised by loss of spatial awareness due to impairment of selective attention. Although the patient has intact peripheral sensation, he ignores novel and meaningful stimuli arising in the space contralateral to the side of the brain.

Patients with unilateral hemispatial sensory neglect (UHN) ignore stimuli (visual, auditory or tactile) arising in relation to their body (body-centred neglect) or in relation to the objects in the neglected hemispace (object-centred neglect).

Several phenomena are associated with UHN. These include anosognosia for hemiplegia (denial of the effects of hemiplegia on the patient's ability to perform motor tasks), anosodiaphoria (indifference to the illness) and kinaesthetic hallucinations (imaginary limb movements). Occasionally patients also report supernumerary (phantom) limbs. The patient is usually alert and has normal cognitive and psychological function.

The occipital cortex

The function of the occipital lobe is the processing and recognition of visual information. Lesions in this part of the cerebral hemisphere cause visual field loss and/or visual perceptual symptoms.

The nature of the visual disturbances due to neurological disease depends largely on the site and size of the brain lesion. Unilateral lesions of the occipital cortex result in congruous (i.e. identical) homonymous hemianopia. However, bilateral lesions cause cortical blindness and are often due to stroke, eclampsia or drug toxicity (e.g. cyclosporine). Cortical blindness is characterised by loss of vision (but the macula may be spared) in the presence of normal pupillary reactions to light. In addition, there is no visual fixation or tracking. Few patients deny blindness and some have visual hallucinations.

Incomplete lesions of the occipital cortex or lesions of the parieto-occipital area usually cause disturbances of visual perception. Rarely, patients with occipital lobe lesions and intact eyesight may experience difficulties with the recognition of familiar faces (prosopagnosia), naming colours in the absence of colour blindness and in the absence of aphasia (colour agnosia), or inability to identify objects by only looking at them (visual object agnosia). In all cases the agnosia is related only to the visual modality, and face and object recognition are possible through other sensory modalities, i.e. smell, touch or sound. Visual distortions may also be present, for example, objects may seem smaller (micropsia) or bigger (macropsia) than their actual size.

Localisation of the most common lesions of the cerebral cortex is shown in figure 1.1.

Figure 1.1
The syndromes of the main focal cortical lesions

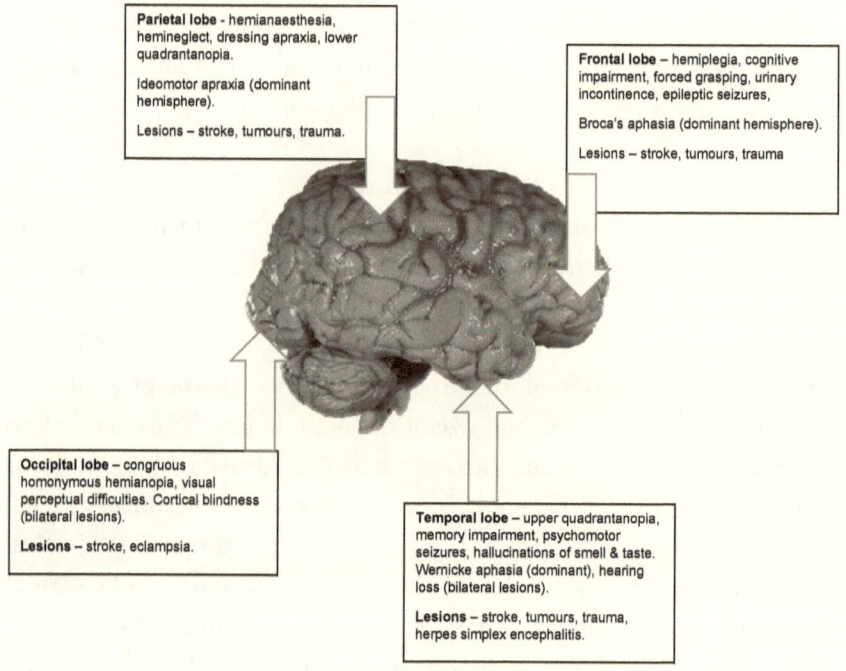

Parietal lobe - hemianaesthesia, hemineglect, dressing apraxia, lower quadrantanopia.

Ideomotor apraxia (dominant hemisphere).

Lesions – stroke, tumours, trauma.

Frontal lobe – hemiplegia, cognitive impairment, forced grasping, urinary incontinence, epileptic seizures,

Broca's aphasia (dominant hemisphere).

Lesions – stroke, tumours, trauma

Occipital lobe – congruous homonymous hemianopia, visual perceptual difficulties. Cortical blindness (bilateral lesions).

Lesions – stroke, eclampsia.

Temporal lobe – upper quadrantanopia, memory impairment, psychomotor seizures, hallucinations of smell & taste. Wernicke aphasia (dominant), hearing loss (bilateral lesions).

Lesions – stroke, tumours, trauma, herpes simplex encephalitis.

4.3 The visual pathways

Certain lesions have predilection for specific parts of the visual pathways and produce typical visual field defects. Basic knowledge of the anatomy of these pathways is essential for the correct localisation of these lesions.

The optic nerve, i.e. the axons of the photoreceptors, runs from the retina under the frontal lobe to the sella turcica. At this point, fibres from the nasal half of the retina of both eyes cross over to the opposite side; thus, forming the optic chiasma. The fibres from the temporal halves of the retina continue uncrossed and join the crossed fibres to form the optic tract. Most of the optic tract fibres terminate in the thalamic nucleus known as the lateral geniculate body. The remaining part of the optic tract terminates in the superior colliculus of the midbrain. The fibres from the lateral geniculate body fan out and travel in the parietal and temporal lobes as the optic radiation then converge and terminate in the occipital lobe (Figure 1.2).

Figure 1.2
Schematic illustration of the visual pathways

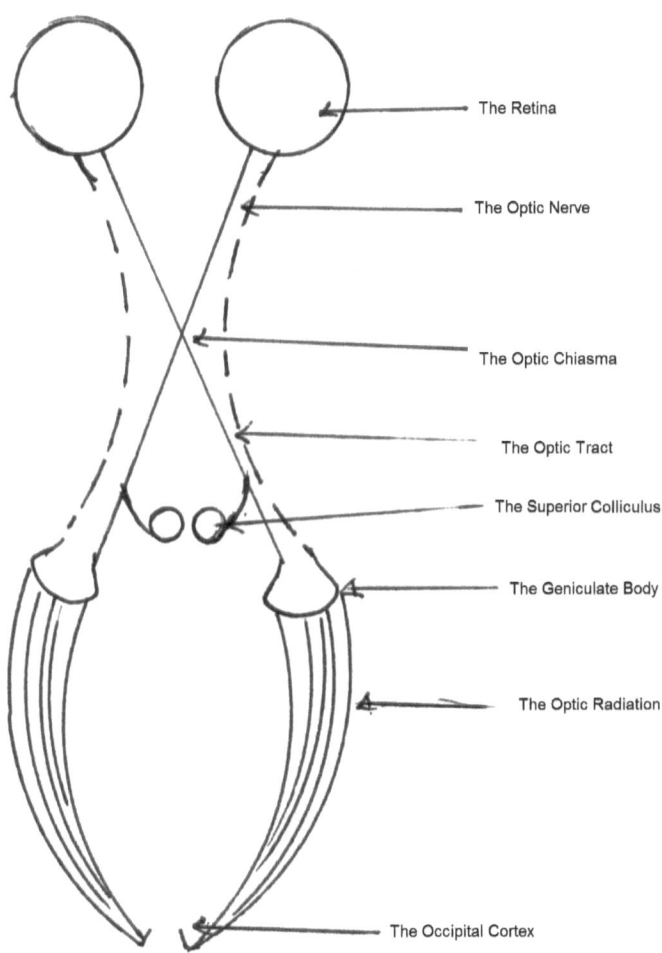

The Retina

The Optic Nerve

The Optic Chiasma

The Optic Tract

The Superior Colliculus

The Geniculate Body

The Optic Radiation

The Occipital Cortex

Lesions of the visual pathways cause various visual field defects (figure 1.3). The visual field loss may affect the nasal half of the retina of both eyes (bitemporal hemianopia), the nasal half of one eye and the temporal half of the other eye (homonymous hemianopia), or a quarter of the field (quadrantanopia). (Note that the visual field defect is opposite to the affected half of the retina.) In some cases, the defect consists in an area of visual field loss surrounded by normal vision. This type of visual field loss is called scotoma.

Complete lesions of the optic nerve cause unilateral blindness and are often due to optic neuritis (e.g. due to multiple sclerosis), drug toxicity (e.g. ethambutol) or a tumour of the anterior cranial fossa. Incomplete optic nerve damage results in central or peripheral scotomas. The effect of a scotoma on vision depends on its site and size. For example, a scotoma in the macula causes severe visual impairment, but a small peripheral scotoma may be completely asymptomatic. The causes of scotomas include multiple sclerosis, nutritional deficiencies, methyl alcohol and some anti-malarial drugs (e.g. chloroquine and quinine).

Damage to the visual pathways at the level of the optic chiasma results in bitemporal hemianopia. Common causes are pituitary adenoma, suprasellar meningioma, internal carotid artery aneurysm and craniopharyngioma.

Optic tract lesions are frequently caused by tuberculous meningitis, syphilis or posterior cerebral artery aneurysms. The typical visual field loss in this case is a homonymous hemianopia. In contrast to the homonymous hemianopia that occurs with a unilateral occipital lobe lesion, the homonymous hemianopia due to optic tract damage is usually incongruous, i.e. the field defect on one side is not identical to that on the other side.

The inferior fibres of the optic radiation are affected by temporal lobe lesions and cause upper quadrantanopia. By contrast, the upper fibres are damaged by parietal lobe lesions and result in lower quadrantanopia.

As described earlier, unilateral lesions of the occipital cortex result in congruous homonymous hemianopia and bilateral lesions cause cortical blindness.

Figure 1.3
Schematic illustration of the common visual field defects

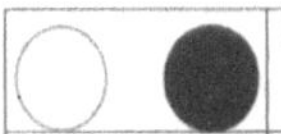	Monocular complete blindness – complete optic nerve lesions.
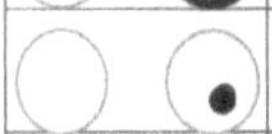	Scotoma – partial optic nerve lesions.
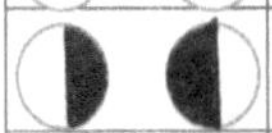	Bitemporal hemianopia – lesions of the optic chiasma.
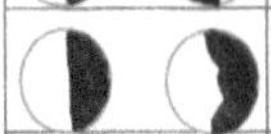	Incongruous homonymous hemianopia – optic tract lesions.
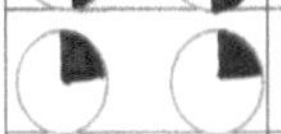	Upper quadrantanopia – lesions of the optic radiation in the temporal lobe.
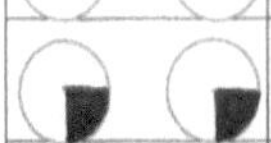	Lower quadrantanopia – lesions of the optic radiation in the parietal lobe.
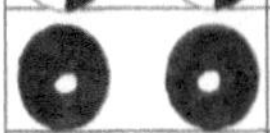	Cortical blindness (macula sparing) – bilateral occipital lobe lesions.
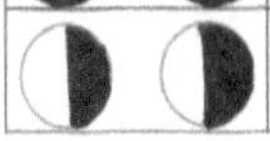	Congruous homonymous hemianopia – unilateral occipital lobe lesions.

4.4 The internal capsule

The internal capsule contains the tightly packed motor fibres of the descending corticospinal and corticobulbar tracts, the ascending sensory fibres from the thalamus to the cerebral cortex and, in its posterior part, the fibres of the optic radiation. The internal capsule lies between the thalamus and the lentiform nucleus. A complete lesion in this area results in hemiplegia, hemianaesthesia and homonymous hemianopia contralateral to the lesion. The most common lesion of the internal capsule is stroke due to middle cerebral artery occlusion or haemorrhage.

4.5 The cranial nerves

Lesions of the cranial nerves can be either isolated (e.g. optic neuritis, Bell's palsy), multiple (e.g. third, fourth and sixth nerve palsy due to retro-orbital tumours) or part of a clinical syndrome, such as Weber syndrome (third nerve palsy and hemiplegia on the contralateral side due to brain stem stroke).

The olfactory nerve (I) – is responsible for the sense of smell. Its fibres arise in the cribriform plate of the ethmoid bone, continue to the olfactory bulb below the frontal lobe and terminate in the temporal lobe. Lesions of the olfactory nerve cause anosmia (loss of the sense of smell). The most frequent neurological causes of anosmia are facial and head injuries, basal meningitis and tumours of the anterior cranial fossa.

The optic nerve (II) – conveys visual perception to the occipital cortex. It also contains the afferent fibres of the light reflex. (The efferent, i.e. motor, fibres are part of the oculomotor nerve.) Lesions of the optic nerve cause complete blindness or scotomas.

The oculomotor nerve (III) – innervates all extraocular muscles except the superior oblique and lateral rectus. It also innervates the levator palpebrae superioris muscle and contains the fibres of the efferent part of the light reflex.

Lesions of the oculomotor nerve result in double vision in all directions except lateral gaze, divergent strabismus (squint), ptosis, a dilated pupil and an absent direct light reflex. Common causes of isolated oculomotor nerve palsy are diabetes mellitus, internal carotid artery aneurysm, ischaemic neuropathy, syphilis, and tentorial herniation due to raised intracranial pressure. The nerve may also be damaged together with other neural structures in the brain stem (due to stroke, multiple sclerosis or brain stem malignant gliomas), in the skull base (basal meningitis), the cavernous sinus (thrombosis) or the petrous temporal bone (middle ear infection).

The trochlear nerve (IV) – innervates the superior oblique muscle. It causes double vision on looking down and to the side opposite to the affected eye, e.g. when reading. Isolated lesions are usually due to facial injuries.

The trigeminal nerve (V) – is a mixed nerve. Its sensory division supplies fibres to part of the scalp and to the facial skin. It also provides the afferent fibres of the corneal reflex. The motor division innervates the muscles of mastication. Unilateral lesions of the trigeminal nerve result in lateral deviation of the jaw. With bilateral lesions, the patient is unable to close his mouth due to weakness of the masseters. (The masseters elevate the jaw.)

Lesions of the trigeminal nerve result from skull fractures, middle ear infections, acoustic neuromas and meningiomas. Other lesions of the trigeminal nerve are herpes zoster and trigeminal neuralgia.

Trigeminal neuralgia
Trigeminal neuralgia is a common cause of facial pain due to neurological disease. It is rare before the age of 40 years and its incidence increases with age. The precise cause of trigeminal neuralgia is not known, but it is thought to be due to compression of the trigeminal nerve by an arteriovenous malformation or an abnormal artery or vein. A family history of trigeminal neuralgia is present in some cases. Patients with multiple sclerosis (MS) appear to have an increased propensity to develop trigeminal neuralgia.

The pain of trigeminal neuralgia is typical. It usually affects one side of the face and occurs in the distribution of at least one of the sensory divisions of the trigeminal nerve. Bilateral facial pain is very rare (it occurs in approximately 5% of patients). The pain is paroxysmal, shock-like and does not radiate. It is brief and lasts a few seconds to a maximum of two minutes. Neurological examination is completely normal (except when trigeminal neuralgia occurs in a patient with MS or other coincidental neurological disorder). Treatment is with carbamazepine or oxcarbazepine. Botulinum toxin injections are also an effective treatment. Surgery should be considered in severe cases that are refractory to medical treatment.

The abducens nerve (VI) – innervates the lateral rectus. It causes double vision on lateral gaze and a convergent squint (the eye is pulled inwards, i.e. towards the nose, by the unopposed action of the medial rectus muscle). Isolated lesions of this nerve usually result from raised intracranial pressure or basal meningitis. Abducens nerve palsy also occurs with lesions of the orbital apex (together with the other oculomotor nerves and the first division of the trigeminal nerve) and with cerebellopontine angle lesions.

The facial nerve (VII) – innervates the facial muscles. The upper half of the nucleus of this nerve receives corticobulbar fibres from both hemispheres. Consequently, a unilateral lesion of the corticobulbar fibres (as often occurs in stroke) causes an upper motor neuron facial weakness, which spares the muscles of the upper half of the face. By contrast, lesions of the nucleus or the nerve itself cause a lower motor neuron weakness. In this case, all facial muscles (on one side) are paralysed. Facial palsy may be caused by fractures of the temporal bone, otitis media and herpes zoster infection (Ramsay Hunt syndrome). However, the most common lower motor neuron lesion of the facial nerve is Bell's palsy.

Bell's palsy

Bell's palsy is the most common cause of acute unilateral lower motor neuron facial weakness. It accounts for approximately 80% of all cases. Its aetiology is not known. The onset is sudden and the muscle weakness is usually complete within a few hours. The clinical features consist of facial asymmetry, the nasolabial fold and the forehead wrinkles on the affected side are smoothed out, and there is unilateral drooping of the angle of the mouth and widening of the palpebral fissure. Voluntary contractions of the facial muscles are weak or absent. For example, the patient is unable to close his eye or to whistle.

Brain imaging or other investigations are usually not necessary. In most cases, spontaneous recovery occurs in approximately 3 weeks, but treatment with corticosteroids (if started within the first 72 hours of onset) shortens the duration of the illness. Taping the eyelid and the use of artificial tears are usually needed to protect against corneal ulceration.

The vestibulocochlear nerve (VIII) – the function of the vestibulocochlear (also called auditory) nerve is hearing and the maintenance of balance. The nerve can be affected by peripheral or central (brain stem) lesions. Disorders of this nerve cause vertigo, vomiting, tinnitus, sensorineural hearing loss and nystagmus.

The most common peripheral lesions are labyrinthitis (vestibular neuronitis) and Ménèire's disease. Ménèire's disease is characterised by intermittent vertigo usually lasting 10 minutes or more, vomiting, tinnitus, nystagmus and progressive sensorineural deafness.

Acute central lesions include stroke in the territory of the posterior inferior cerebellar artery, aura of an epileptic seizure and migraine aura. Slowly evolving symptoms usually result from brain stem tumours.

The glossopharyngeal (IX), vagus (X) and the spinal accessory nerves (XI) – the glossopharyngeal nerve innervates the pharyngeal muscles and, in addition, supplies sensory fibres to the pharyngeal wall. The vagus innervates the soft palate and the internal organs. The spinal accessory is a motor nerve to the sternomastoid and trapezius muscles. These nerves are considered together because individually they are very rarely affected by injury or disease. However, together they may be damaged by posterior fossa tumours, metastases or a basilar artery aneurysm resulting in the so-called jagular foramen syndrome.

The clinical features of the jagular foramen syndrome are dysphonia and a hoarse voice (due to vocal cord paralysis), dysphagia, nasal regurgitation of fluids, deviation of the soft palate to the unaffected side, sensory loss in the pharyngeal wall, and weakness of the sternomastoid and trapezius muscles.

The hypoglossal nerve (XII)
The hypoglossal nerve is the motor nerve to the tongue. Lesions affecting the nerve (e.g. neurofibromas) or its nucleus (e.g. bulbar poliomyelitis) cause a lower motor tongue weakness: the tongue is atrophic, flaccid and deviated to the affected side, and the tongue movements are weak. Fasciculations (visible twitching of the muscle fibres) may be present. Supra nuclear lesions (in the corticobulbar tract) result in an upper motor neuron tongue weakness. In these cases, the tongue looks small and pointed (because of the increase in muscle tone) and the tongue movements are weak. The jaw jerk is exaggerated. The causes of hypoglossal nerve palsy include motor neurone disease, basal meningitis, granulomas and tumours.

4.6 The basal ganglia
The basal ganglia is a group of large subcortical nuclei that include the caudate nucleus and putamen (the two together are called the corpus striatum or striatum), the globus pallidus (or pallidum), the substantia nigra and the subthalamic nucleus. These structures have an important

role in the control of voluntary movements and posture, muscle tone, behaviour, emotions and motivation.

Diseases of the basal ganglia cause numerous symptoms and signs, including tremor, chorea (involuntary, purposeless jerky limb movements), athetosis (similar to chorea but the movements are slow), dystonia (described in Chapter 7), myoclonus (brief, shock-like involuntary movements), bradykinesia (slowness of movements), abnormalities of gait and posture, and poor motivation.

Parkinson's disease is the most common disease of the basal ganglia. It is due to degenerative changes of unknown cause that occur mainly in the substantia nigra. Treatment with phenothiazines, butyrophenones (e.g. haloperidol) and other drugs also causes basal ganglia disease. Other lesions of the basal ganglia include spontaneous intracerebral haemorrhage, arteriovenous malformations, metabolic disorders, e.g. severe hypoglycaemia, and trauma. Primary basal ganglia tumours are rare.

4.7 The brain stem

The structures that are collectively referred to as the brain stem are the medulla, pons, midbrain, the cerebral aqueduct and the fourth ventricle. The brain stem contains the nuclei of the cranial nerves, the reticular formation, the descending motor pathways and the ascending sensory fibres. In addition, it has an important role in the regulation of cardiac and respiratory function, consciousness, arousal and the sleep-wake cycle.

Large lesions of the brain stem are incompatible with life and result in death. Small, discrete lesions cause a variety of signs and clinical syndromes depending on the site and size of the lesion. The syndromes include bulbar and pseudobulbar palsy, the locked-in syndrome, the crossed brain stem syndromes and disorders of conjugate gaze. The main causes of brain stem disease are stroke, multiple sclerosis, primary and metastatic tumours, motor neurone disease and trauma.

The syndrome of bulbar palsy

Bulbar palsy is due to medullary lesions that affect the nuclei of the glossopharyngeal, vagus, spinal accessory and hypoglossal nerves. The patient presents with dysphonia, dysphagia, nasal regurgitation of fluids and dysarthria. On examination, the soft palate does not move on phonation; tongue fasciculations are present; and the tongue is flaccid, atrophic and weak. The sternomastoid and trapezius muscles are also weak. The jaw jerk is depressed or absent.

The syndrome of pseudobulbar palsy

Pseudobulbar palsy is an upper motor neuron syndrome that involves the corticobulbar tracts. It results from damage to the fibres that connect the frontal lobe motor neurons to the nuclei of the IX, X, XI and XII nerves. The symptoms are similar to those of bulbar palsy, but the tongue is spastic, there is no fasciculations or atrophy and the jaw jerk is exaggerated.

The crossed brain stem syndromes

These are characterised by a lower motor neuron lesion of a cranial nerve and hemiplegia on the opposite side of the body. (The corticospinal tract in the brain stem runs in close proximity to the nuclei of some of the cranial nerves.) An example of the crossed brain stem syndromes is Weber syndrome, which results from stroke and consists of oculomotor nerve palsy and contralateral hemiplegia.

The locked-in syndrome

This syndrome is due to destruction of the corticospinal tracts and the ascending sensory pathways in the midbrain. It usually results from basilar artery stroke or traumatic brain injury. The patient is quadriplegic and mute (due to anarhria). However, voluntary vertical eye movements and eyelid movements are intact. Intellectual function (including language function) and the normal sleep-wake cycles are preserved.

Abnormalities of conjugate gaze

Conjugate gaze is the coordinated simultaneous movement of both eyes in the same direction. It is regulated by neurons in the pontine reticular formation, and the frontal and occipital lobes. Impulses from these structures are transmitted via the medial longitudinal bundle to the nuclei of the fourth and sixth cranial nerves. Abnormalities of conjugate lateral gaze may result from lesions of the frontal or occipital lobes, or from pontine lesions. Vertical gaze palsies often arise from pineal tumours and tumours of the splenium of the corpus callosum.

An abnormality of conjugate horizontal eye movements consisting of failure of adduction (i.e. inward movement of the eye ipsilateral to the lesion) and jerk nystagmus of the other eye is known as internuclear ophthalmoplegia. It is due to a lesion in the medial longitudinal bundle and may result from brain stem vascular lesions or tumours, e.g. brain stem glioma. Bilateral internuclear ophthalmoplegia is considered pathognomonic of multiple sclerosis.

4.8 The cerebellum

The main function of the cerebellum is the maintenance of balance and posture and the coordination of goal-directed voluntary movements. Cerebellar disease causes severe limb, trunk and gait ataxia. (Ataxia is the inability to accurately execute goal-directed voluntary movements in the absence of significant muscle weakness, severe abnormality of muscle tone, dyspraxia or involuntary movements of the affected limbs.) Other features of cerebellar disease are vertigo, dysarthria, nystagmus (involuntary jerky eye movements), low muscle tone and reduced tendon reflexes. Mass lesions of the cerebellar midline structures, such as medulloblastomas, can also obstruct the aqueduct of the fourth ventricle and cause hydrocephalus. Very large cerebellar lesions result in skew deviation of the eyes. (Skew deviation is the downward and inward deviation of the eye on the side of the lesion, and upward and outward deviation of the opposite eye. However, the axes of the eyes become parallel on visual fixation.)

Common causes of cerebellar disease are multiple sclerosis, stroke, excessive alcohol consumption, toxicity of antiepileptic drugs (e.g. phenytoin), hereditary degenerative disorders, and tumours. Most tumours of the cerebellum are metastases from the breast, lung or large bowel. Primary cerebellar tumours are rare.

Cerebellopontine angle (CPA) lesions

Certain tumours tend to occur in the CPA. The CPA is formed by the petrous temporal bone, the lateral part of the pons and the cerebellum. It contains the trigeminal, abducens, facial and vestibulocochlear nerves.

The most common tumours of the CPA are acoustic neuromas, meningiomas, and cholesteatomas. Basilar artery aneurysms also occur in the CPA. Tinnitus in one ear, progressive sensorineural deafness and loss of the corneal reflex are the first clinical manifestations of these lesions. Facial palsy, vertigo, sensory loss in the trigeminal nerve dermatomes, and cerebellar and pyramidal tract signs are late features.

4.9 The motor system

The motor system consists of a group of descending pathways that originate mainly in the motor area of the frontal lobes and terminate in the motor nuclei of the cranial nerves (the corticobulbar tracts) or the anterior horn cells, i.e. the alpha motor neurons, of the spinal cord (the corticospinal tracts). The axons of the cranial motor nuclei innervate facial and some neck muscles. The axons of the anterior horn cells emerge from the spinal cord in the anterior (ventral) nerve roots and then divide to form the peripheral motor nerves that innervate skeletal muscles. Other descending fibres, namely the vestibulospinal and reticulospinal tracts, control muscle tone. They run adjacent to the corticospinal tracts. The motor frontal lobe areas also have numerous fibre connections with the basal ganglia, cerebellum and the sensory cortex.

Lesions of the motor system result either in an upper or lower motor neuron syndrome.

The upper motor neuron syndrome

The fibres of the corticospinal (also called pyramidal) tract originate in the precentral gyrus and descend in the posterior limb of the internal capsule down to the midbrain. At the junction of the pons and medulla, most of the fibres cross over to the opposite side and become the lateral corticospinal tract. The uncrossed fibres descend as the anterior (ventral) corticospinal tract. The corticospinal tracts terminate on the spinal alpha motor neurons. Damage to the pyramidal tracts at any point from the cortex to the spinal alpha motor neurons causes an upper motor neuron syndrome. The clinical manifestation of the upper motor neuron syndrome is spastic hemiplegia, paraplegia or tetraplegia depending on the site of the lesion. Hemiplegia is due to a lesion of the descending tracts on one side. By contrast, paraplegia and tetraplegia (also called quadriplegia) are caused by bilateral lesions.

Hemiplegia

Hemiplegia is complete paralysis of the arm and leg opposite to the side of the lesion, whereas hemiparesis is partial paralysis. In cases of hemiparesis, the distal muscles are usually more severely affected than the proximal muscles and the upper limbs are frequently weaker than the lower limbs.

Paraplegia and tetraplegia

Paraplegia and tetraplegia are caused by lesions in the spinal cord or the brain stem. (Occasionally paraplegia is caused by parasagittal frontal lobe lesions.) In addition to the upper motor neuron signs, in paraplegia and tetraplegia there is also loss of all sensory modalities below the level of the lesion and loss of bladder and bowel control. In quadriplegia, destruction of the sympathetic neurons (of the intermediolateral cell column) also results in Horner's syndrome (a small pupil, ptosis, enophthalmos – sunken eyeballs – and absent sweating on half of the face).

Incomplete lesions of the spinal cord that destroy half the spinal segment (known as hemisection of the spinal cord or Brown-Séquard syndrome) are usually associated with spinal cord knife injuries. The lesion may cause spastic hemiplegia or spastic weakness of one leg depending on whether the injury is in the cervical or thoracic region. The limb weakness is ipsilateral to the lesion and is accompanied by loss of proprioceptive and vibration sense on the same side and loss of spinothalamic sensation on the opposite side (see the explanation in the section on the sensory system). Bladder and bowel function is not affected because of the bilateral of innervation of these organs.

The signs of the upper motor neuron syndrome

An upper motor neuron syndrome causes muscle weakness, increased muscle tone (spasticity), exaggerated deep tendon reflexes, sustained ankle clonus, loss of abdominal reflexes and an extensor plantar response (Babinski sign).

The lower motor neuron syndrome

The lower motor neuron consists of the spinal alpha motor neurons and their nerve fibre connections to the skeletal muscles. Lower motor neuron damage causes reduced muscle tone (hypotonia, flaccid muscle tone), muscle weakness, loss of tendon reflexes, focal muscle wasting and fasciculations.

The lower motor neuron syndrome is caused by lesions of the anterior horn neurons, e.g. cell necrosis following poliomyelitis or degeneration due to motor neurone disease, and by disorders of the peripheral nervous system.

Table 1.3

Summary of the clinical features of the upper (UMN) and lower motor neuron (LMN) syndromes:

Clinical symptom or sign	UMN syndrome	LMN syndrome
Muscle weakness	Present	Present
Muscle tone	Increased – spasticity	Reduced – flaccid tone
Muscle atrophy	Absent	Present
Fasciculations	Absent	May be present
Tendon reflexes	Exaggerated	Diminished or absent
Extensor plantar response	Present	Absent

4.10 The sensory system

Sensory impulses from the skin, muscles and joints are conveyed to the brain by two routes. The fibres that carry the sensations of light touch, temperature and pain are contained in the sensory and sensorimotor nerves and the posterior nerve roots. They enter the spinal cord and cross over to the opposite side just anterior to the spinal canal. Then they ascend the spinal cord in the lateral column and continue in the brain stem to the thalamus. This sensory pathway is known as the spinothalamic tract.

Sensory feedback from skeletal muscles and joints, i.e. proprioceptive sense, also reaches the spinal cord via the peripheral nerves and the posterior nerve roots. In the spinal cord, these fibres continue in the posterior columns and terminate in the medulla on the gracile and cuneate nuclei. The axons from these nuclei cross to the opposite side and ascend to the thalamus as the medial lemniscus. From the thalamus, all sensory fibres continue their ascent together through the internal capsule to the primary sensory area of the parietal lobe.

Some patients present with predominantly sensory symptoms, and localisation of the lesion that is responsible for the symptoms often helps in identifying the underlying pathology (figure 1.4). Loss or impairment of all sensory modalities occurs with lesions of the sensory peripheral nerves, the upper brain stem and the internal capsule. Lesions that expand the spinal canal, such as ependymomas and syringomyelia, destroy the spinothalamic fibres as they cross to the opposite side. Thus, they cause spinothalamic sensory loss at the level of the lesion, but spare the posterior column sensation. (Syringomyelia is characterised by cavity formation in the spinal canal, usually in the cervical region. Most frequently it is due to congenital abnormalities, such as Arnold Chiari malformation. In some patients it is caused by intramedullary tumours.) In contrast to lesions of the spinothalamic pathways, disorders of the posterior columns (e.g. subacute combined degeneration of the spinal cord) cause loss of proprioceptive sense, while touch, temperature and pain sensation remain intact.

Figure 1.4
The sensory pathways

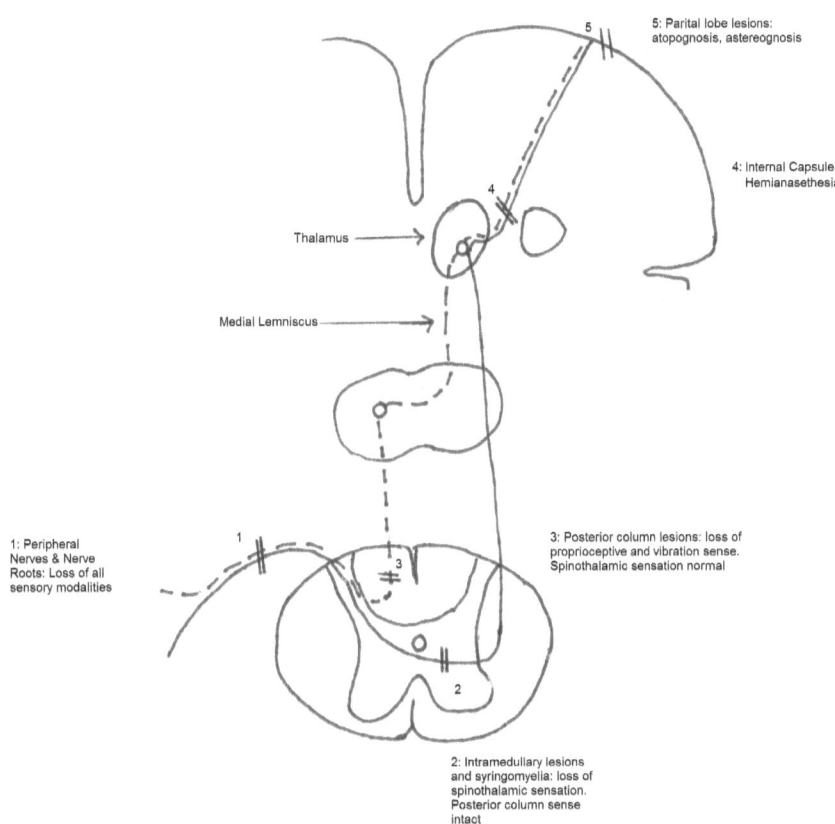

5: Parital lobe lesions:
atopognosis, astereognosis

4: Internal Capsule:
Hemianasethesia

Thalamus

Medial Lemniscus

1: Peripheral
Nerves & Nerve
Roots: Loss of all
sensory modalities

3: Posterior column lesions: loss of
proprioceptive and vibration sense.
Spinothalamic sensation normal

2: Intramedullary lesions
and syringomyelia: loss of
spinothalamic sensation.
Posterior column sense
intact

4.11 The spinal cord

The main causes of the spinal cord syndromes are trauma, severe cervical spondylosis, intraspinal extramedullary or intramedullary tumours, metastasis of malignant tumours, transverse myelitis associated with multiple sclerosis or viral infections, epidural abscess and vertebral osteomyelitis.

Spinal pathology may selectively involve a specific structure of the spinal cord and spare the rest, as occurs with selective necrosis of the anterior horn cells in poliomyelitis. Alternatively, it may affect the whole segment or a number of segments, e.g. in transverse myelitis. Any level of the spinal cord can be affected and some conditions have predilection for certain parts. For example, meningiomas are usually found in the thoracic region, whereas chordomas tend to occur in the sacral spinal cord. Therefore, spinal cord disease can cause various clinical syndromes depending on the nature and location of the lesion, and on whether the cord involvement is complete or partial. Paraplegia, tetraplegia and hemisection of the spinal cord were described earlier. Other spinal cord syndromes are the conus medullaris and cauda equina syndromes.

The conus medullaris syndrome
The conus medullaris syndrome results from damage to the terminal part of the spinal cord. It causes sensory loss around the anus and in the posterior part of the thigh (which is often referred to as saddle anaesthesia); an areflexic, hypotonic bladder and bowel; and loss of penile erection. The ankle jerk is present when the first sacral root (S1) is spared. Partial lesions may cause priapism. (Priapism is usually defined as continuous, painful erection of the penis that lasts four hours or more.)

The cauda equina syndrome
The clinical features of the cauda equina syndrome are indistinguishable from those of the conus medullaris syndrome, except that the sensory symptoms are more extensive and there is also a lower motor neuron weakness in the lower limbs (which is usually asymmetrical). The cauda equina syndrome is due to lesions of the lumbosacral roots within the spinal canal, e.g. metastatic tumours.

Bladder and bowel dysfunction due to spinal cord lesions
The initiation of micturition and the maintenance of continence are regulated by neurons in the medial aspect of the frontal lobes. The axons of these cells descend as part of the spinoreticular, and the medial and anterior reticulospinal tracts. The first two tracts convey neural impulses that initiate micturition. The spinoreticular tract facilitates contraction of the detrusor muscle and relaxation of the urethral sphincter. The anterior reticulospinal tract inhibits the detrusor muscle and causes the urethral sphincter to contract. Damage to the corticospinal pathways often leads to involuntary contractions of the detrusor muscle during bladder filling. This

is known as detrusor hyperreflexia and is the main type of incontinence that occurs as a direct result of an upper motor neuron lesion. Detrusor hyperreflexia is caused by damage to the sacral nerve roots.

In a small number of patients, the detrusor muscle contraction is not accompanied by the coordinated relaxation of the urethral sphincter, a condition known as detrusor-sphincter dyssynergia. It is common in patients with spinal cord injury.

4.12 The peripheral nervous system and muscle

The components of the peripheral nervous system are the autonomic nervous system, the cranial nerves (except the optic), the spinal nerves, the neuromuscular junction and the sensory receptors.

The autonomic nervous system

The autonomic nervous system innervates the glands and the smooth muscle of internal organs. Together with the endocrine system it regulates the function of the cardiovascular, respiratory and digestive systems, as well as sexual function. It also controls the pupillary reactions and bowel and bladder function.

The autonomic nervous system consists of two parts: the sympathetic and the parasympathetic systems. Its function is regulated by the hypothalamus and neurons in the brain stem. Stimulation of the sympathetic system causes pupillary dilatation, tachycardia, bronchodilation, excessive sweating, vasoconstriction and piloerection. Stimulation of the parasympathetic system has the opposite effect. Each of the sympathetic and parasympathetic pathways has two neurons: preganglionic and ganglionic. Postganglionic fibres innervate the target organ.

The preganglionic neurons of the sympathetic system are housed in the lateral horn of the spinal cord from T1 to L2 segments. The axons of these neurons join the anterior nerve roots and terminate in the cervical, thoracic, lumbar, sacral and coccygeal paravertebral ganglia. The ganglia are joined together to form the sympathetic chain. Some fibres from the cervical ganglia and from the first and second thoracic spinal cord segments (T1 and T2) ascend the carotid arteries to the orbit and innervate the ciliary muscle and the constrictor of the pupil. Damage to these fibres causes Horner's syndrome.

The fibres of the parasympathetic system arise from the nuclei of the oculomotor, facial, glossopharyngeal and vagus nerves, and also from neurons in the second, third and fourth sacral segments of the spinal cord (S2-S4). They send their axons to ganglia in, or adjacent to their target organs, e.g. the ciliary muscle, the sphincter of the pupil, the salivary glands or the viscera.

Lesions of the sympathetic or parasympathetic systems occur either in the brain stem (e.g. poliomyelitis, multiple sclerosis, tumours) or in any part of their fibre pathways (tumours of the lung apex or neck, high spinal cord injuries, transverse myelitis, Guillain-Barré syndrome, etc.). Systemic disease, e.g. diabetes mellitus and alcohol abuse, may also cause partial or total failure of the autonomic function.

The clinical features of autonomic nervous system dysfunction are severe hypotension, anhidrosis, constipation, dry mouth, dry eyes, loss of libido, impotence and loss of pupillary reflexes.

The spinal nerves
Motor and sensory axons leave each segment of the spinal cord in the anterior and posterior nerve roots, respectively. Then they join together to form a spinal nerve. In total there are 31 pairs of spinal nerves. The first four spinal nerves (which arise from the first four cervical segments, C1-C4) innervate the occipital and some neck muscles. The remaining spinal nerves form the brachial plexus (C5-8), the thoracic spinal nerves (T1-12), the lumbar (L1-5) and sacral plexuses (S1-5), and one coccygeal nerve. The thoracic spinal nerves innervate the intercostal and trunk muscles. The spinal nerves also have sensory fibres. Each spinal nerve supplies a separate skin area, i.e. a dermatome.

The brachial plexus innervates the muscles and skin of the upper limbs and some of the neck muscles. The most common cause of brachial plexus damage is trauma (e.g. motor cycle accidents). Brachial neuritis and neurofibromas are other causes. The patient complains of severe neuropathic pain, numbness and dysaesthesia in the upper limbs. Physical examination reveals skin sensory loss, muscle weakness, and wasting and loss of the upper limb tendon reflexes.

The lumbosacral plexus innervates the skin and muscles of the abdominal wall and lower limbs. The most common disorders of the lumbosacral plexus are diabetic amyotrophy (also called diabetic lumbosacral plexopathy), tumours (e.g. colorectal carcinoma, metastatic breast tumours) and obstetric complications. Lumbosacral plexus lesions cause neuropathic pain in the lumbar region, buttocks and thighs, and also patchy sensory loss that does not fit the dermatomal distribution of a single nerve root or a peripheral nerve. They also cause progressive lower limb weakness and wasting, loss of tendon reflexes and incontinence of bowel and bladder.

A more detailed description of the common disorders of the peripheral nervous system is provided in Chapter 11.

Muscle diseases
Muscle diseases include inflammatory myopathies (polymyositis, dermatomyositis, polymyalgia rheumatica), drug-induced myopathies (steroids), hereditary muscular dystrophies, disorders of neuromuscular transmission (e.g. myasthenia gravis) and tumours (rhabdomyoma, rhabdomyosarcoma).

The common clinical features of muscle disease are myalgia (muscle pain), muscle weakness and wasting, and reduced muscle tone. Occasionally the weak muscles are increased in size (rather than atrophic), as in Duchene's muscular dystrophy. Rarely, the main symptom is delayed muscle relaxation (myotonia). The medical and family history, the presence of other clinical symptoms and signs, the distribution of muscle weakness (focal or generalised) and laboratory tests help to distinguish these clinical entities.

5. The differential diagnosis

A neurological disease may be congenital, hereditary or, more often, acquired. It can be caused by vascular lesions, infections, immune disorders, trauma or tumours, and metabolic and endocrine disorders.

In addition to the medical and family history, the mode of onset, the evolution of the symptoms and the course of the disease, as well as the findings of the neurological examination and the tendency of certain disorders to occur in specific sites all provide important clues that often enable a differential diagnosis.

Neurological symptoms and signs that occur suddenly and evolve quickly are usually due to vascular events. By contrast, an acute onset and progression of the symptoms over several hours suggest central nervous system (CNS) infection, systemic sepsis or severe metabolic disorders, and, invariably, in these cases there is additional clinical evidence of systemic disease, e.g. high fever, a source of infection, etc. Gradual onset of symptoms and slow evolution and the presence of focal neurological signs usually suggest a tumour as the underlying pathological cause. Confirmation of the provisional clinical diagnosis is made with objective laboratory tests.

6. Laboratory confirmation of the clinical diagnosis

The selection of a neurological laboratory test depends on the type of the suspected pathology. For example, brain imaging is used for the detection of structural lesions; electroencephalography is invaluable for the investigation of patients presenting with episodic loss of consciousness; electromyography is often useful for the differentiation between various muscle and peripheral nerve diseases; and serological tests or culture of the cerebrospinal fluid can provide definitive confirmation of CNS infection. In addition to the specialist neurological investigations, tests such as full blood count, renal and liver function tests, etc. can provide evidence of systemic (non-neurological) disease.

6.1 Imaging of the nervous system

Computerised tomographic (CT) scans, magnetic resonance imaging (MRI) scans, ultrasound and angiography are widely used to confirm the diagnosis of structural lesions of the nervous system and in monitoring the course of the disease or the effects of treatment.

CT scan images are produced from numerous X-ray pictures taken from different angles and processed by computer to form cross-sectional images. Therefore, in contrast to MRI, they expose the patient to radiation. Nonetheless, because they have good spatial resolution and are less costly than MRI scans they are considered the first choice investigation of CNS structural lesions. Additional diagnostic information can be obtained by the use of a contrast medium, e.g. a gadolinium-based agent, with a CT or MRI.

MRI scans are superior to CT scans in the evaluation of posterior fossa and spinal cord lesions. T1-weighted MRI scan images give high spatial resolution, while T2-weighted images give better contrast resolution and are particularly useful for the detection of inflammation, oedema and demyelination. Magnetic resonance angiography (MRA) is useful in the diagnosis of vascular pathology (arterial stenosis, aneurysms, etc.). Various modifications of MRI techniques are also used in clinical practice, e.g. for the early diagnosis of ischaemic stroke (diffusion MRI), or to improve the detection rate of lesions in the periventricular brain areas by suppressing the effect of CSF signals (fluid attenuation inversion recovery images – FLAIR). In addition to its use in the diagnosis of structural lesions, MRI is used in research to study cognitive function by measuring the activation of different neuronal populations during a functional task. This is known as functional magnetic resonance imaging (fMRI). The contraindications to MRI are implanted electric devices, such as cardiac pacemakers and cochlear implants, and metallic foreign bodies.

Ultrasound is particularly useful because of its low cost, but its diagnostic accuracy depends on the experience of the operator. The main value of ultrasound is in the diagnosis of peripheral nervous system lesions, such as entrapment neuropathies and tumours of nerves and muscle.

6.2 Examination of the cerebrospinal fluid

Examination of the cerebrospinal fluid (CSF) is an essential part of the diagnostic workup of many neurological disorders, especially CNS infections and inflammatory diseases. Analysis of the CSF protein, glucose and cell content yields useful diagnostic information. Serological and microbiology tests are also useful in many cases. The CSF samples are, as a rule, obtained by lumbar puncture.

The lumber puncture (LP)

The LP is carried out with the patient sitting up or, preferably, lying down. If the recumbent position is chosen, the patient should lie on his side with his neck, hips and knees maximally flexed. The site of needle insertion is marked. This is the intervertebral disc space between L2-L3 or L3-L4. The skin is then cleansed with an antiseptic solution, and the skin and deep tissues are infiltrated with a local anaesthetic. A 22 gauge (or 25 gauge if the patient is thin) bevel lumbar puncture needle is introduced 4-5 cm before the stylet is removed to allow the free flow of CSF. Measurement of the CSF pressure is performed by attaching the LP needle to a manometer. (The patient's legs should be extended during the measurement as hip and knee flexion increase CSF pressure and result in an incorrect reading.) Following the procedure, the patient should be encouraged to drink plenty of fluids and to remain in bed for a few hours to prevent post-LP headache. LP is contraindicated if an intracranial space-occupying lesion is present. In doubtful cases, a CT head scan should be carried out before the LP. Other contraindications are the presence of skin infection at the LP site and blood clotting disorders.

The normal CSF is clear and colourless. It contains 0-4 lymphocytes per cubic millilitre, 15-50 mg/dL of protein and 45-80 mg/dL of glucose. The normal LP opening CSF pressure is 65-195 mmHg.

Increase in the number of CSF cells (pleocytosis) is found in many disorders. Lymphocytic pleocytosis suggests viral infections or an inflammatory disease. On the other hand, neutrophil pleocytosis occurs with bacterial infections. Changes in the glucose and protein content also have a diagnostic significance and are discussed in the relevant chapters of this book. In some cases, additional diagnostic information can be obtained from CSF protein electrophoresis. For example, oligoclonal bands (IgG) are often present in multiple sclerosis, Guillain-Barré syndrome, Lyme disease, neurosarcoidosis and neurosyphilis.

6.3 Electroencephalography

Electroencephalography is a non-invasive method of recording the brain's electrical activity with surface electrodes placed on the scalp according to a standardised protocol. (Intracranial recording is also used in some cases, e.g. in the surgical treatment of epilepsy.) It is a valuable test for the confirmation of epilepsy, the type of seizure and the site of the epileptogenic focus. (The EEG abnormalities in epilepsy are discussed in Chapter 3.) It is also useful in sleep studies, the diagnosis of brain death, encephalopathies and other brain pathology.

The routine electroencephalogram (EEG) is recorded with the patient resting comfortably on a couch. In some cases, e.g. in the diagnosis of pseudoseizures, it is also recorded in ambulatory subjects and may be combined with video recording (EEG video telemetry). Some procedures, such as recording during natural or drug-induced sleep, stimulation with flashing lights, or hyperventilation, are used to activate latent abnormalities.

Four types of waves are distinguishable in the EEG: alpha, beta, delta and theta. They differ in their frequency (periodicity as measured in cycles per second or hertz – Hz), shape, site and how they are affected by the subject's state of alertness during the recording. In a healthy adult, alpha rhythm (frequency 8-14 Hz) is recorded from the occipital region when the subject is relaxed and his eyes are closed. Beta waves (14 Hz or more) are recorded from the frontal and temporal areas when the subject is alert and thinking. Delta (less than 4 Hz) and theta (4-7 Hz) are present during sleep and are recorded from the frontal brain regions.

6.4 Electromyography and nerve conduction studies

Electromyography (EMG) and nerve conduction studies (NCS) are used in the diagnosis of diseases of the neuromuscular junction, muscles and peripheral nerves.

EMG measures, either with surface or needle electrodes, the electrical activity generated in skeletal muscles. Needle EMG is usually used for diagnostic purposes. The muscle activity is recorded at rest and during maximal voluntary contraction. Although insertion of the EMG needle into the muscle produces electrical (insertional) activity, once the needle is in place no action potential is recordable from a resting healthy muscle. Approximately 90% of the action potentials of a healthy muscle are triphasic and the remaining 10% are polyphasic. Increase in the number of the triphasic potentials and the occurrence of spontaneous activity in a resting muscle (fibrillation potentials and positive sharp waves) indicate muscle denervation or an inflammatory myopathy. In cases of muscle denervation, the amplitude of the action potential is also reduced. Giant waves (due to partial reinnervation) may also be present in cases of chronic denervation. Significant increase in the insertional activity typically occurs in myopathies.

NCS consist of placing two electrodes on different points along a peripheral nerve, stimulation of the nerve at one site, and recording the latency (i.e. the time from the stimulus to the start of the action potential) and the conduction velocity at the other site. The wave shape and amplitude are also recorded. NCS are used for the diagnosis of motor and sensory neuropathies and radiculopathies.

6.5 Visual and somatosensory evoked responses

Visual evoked responses (VERs) measure nerve conduction in the visual pathways. The optic nerve is stimulated with a light stimulus (a flickering checkerboard pattern), and the latency and the conduction velocity are recorded over the occipital cortex. A long latency, reduced conduction velocity (normal value 120 msec) and low amplitude are signs of disorders of the optic nerve or optic tracts. The test is very sensitive. For example in multiple sclerosis, changes in VERs usually precede any clinically detectable abnormalities of visual acuity, colour vision or signs of optic neuritis on fundoscopy.

Sensory evoked responses are also used for measuring conduction in the auditory pathways (auditory evoked responses) by applying a sound stimulus to the ear and recording over the scalp. Similarly, sensory conduction along nerve roots and peripheral nerves can be evaluated with somatosensory evoked potentials and is useful in the diagnosis of radiculopathies and peripheral nerve injuries.

6.6 Biopsy of neural tissue and muscle

Biopsy of neural tissues is indicated when the results of non-invasive investigations are equivocal and a definitive diagnosis cannot be made otherwise. Either open or needle biopsy may be used. Biopsy of malignant tumours provides histological diagnosis and prognostic information and helps with treatment selection. Nerve biopsy (usually of the sural or superficial peroneal nerve) is especially valuable in the diagnosis of neuropathies due to vasculitis, sarcoidosis, Lyme disease and human deficiency virus infection. Muscle biopsy is indicated for the definitive diagnosis of myopathies.

CHAPTER 2

MANAGEMENT OF COMMON
NEUROLOGICAL IMPAIRMENTS

The main physical impairments due to neurological disease are dysphasia, dysarthria, dyspraxia, unilateral hemispatial neglect, visual impairment, impairment of cognitive function, muscle weakness, ataxia, dysphagia, mood disorders, and bladder and bowel dysfunction. These impairments occur in various combinations depending on the site and size of the underlying lesion. They often persist and cause significant functional disability even after the successful treatment of the primary neurological disease. The appropriate management of these impairments is an important part of the medical treatment of most patients with neurological disorders.

Assessment and management of dysphasia

Dysphasia is one of the most common focal neurological deficits. It is broadly classified into predominantly expressive (motor, Broca's dysphasia) or predominantly receptive type (sensory, Wernicke's dysphasia). In the assessment of dysphasia, it is important to establish the patient's handedness and to determine the type and severity of the language impairment.

Assessment of handedness

The hemisphere where the neurons responsible for language function are located is called the dominant hemisphere. There is a strong correlation between lateralisation of language function to the left hemisphere and the person's preference to use his right hand in tasks that require the use of only one hand, such as cutting with a knife or throwing a ball. Therefore, establishing the patient's hand preference (or handedness) may be used as a simple method for determining cerebral hemisphere dominance.

Different methods have been devised to assess handedness. For routine clinical practice it is probably sufficient to determine handedness by recording the patient's responses to the following five questions: which hand they prefer to use to throw a ball, hold a toothbrush, cut bread, hold a spoon and strike a match. Hand preference for writing and drawing should not be used as it is often influenced by cultural norms. Left-handedness tends to run in families, so a family history of left-handedness is also helpful in the diagnosis.

Assessment of the language deficit
The language deficit in dysphasia may involve any component of the linguistic system, i.e. the phonological (sounds that form words), morphological-lexical (word form), syntactic (grammar) or semantic component (word meaning). In all, but mild cases, the rate and rhythm of the patient's verbal output are frequently disrupted and the speech may contain paraphasic errors. (In paraphasia, letters in a word may be omitted, added or substituted, or a word may be replaced by a conceptually similar one, e.g. chair for stool, or pen for pencil.) In addition, the construction of the sentences may become grammatically incorrect (agrammatism). In very mild dysphasia the language impairment may consist of only word-finding difficulties (anomia).

Expressive dysphasia is characterised by reduced verbal fluency. The speech is sparse and in severe cases it is completely or almost completely absent. Interestingly, well-learnt phrases such as prayers and emotional language, e.g. swearing, are often preserved. Language comprehension is not affected and the patient usually has insight into his disability and is often frustrated by it. Depression is common in these patients. Some dysphasic patients produce stereotyped utterances. These may be correct words or non-words that are repeated several times whenever the patient attempts to speak. Dysprosody is also common and is characterised by slow, monotonous speech (table 2.1).

In receptive dysphasia the deficit is primarily that of language comprehension. Verbal fluency is usually increased in receptive dysphasia. Paraphasias are common. Sometimes patients invent new words that did not exist in their language (neologism). When paraphasia, agrammatism and neologism are present together, the patient is said to have jargon dysphasia.

Table 2.1
The salient features of expressive and receptive dysphasia:

Expressive (Broca's) dysphasia	Receptive (Wernicke's) dysphasia
1. Non-fluent	1. Fluent
2. Language comprehension not affected	2. Poor language comprehension
3. Insight into deficit retained	3. No insight
4. Dysprosody	4. Paraphasias are common
5. Frustration and depression are common	5. Jargon dysphasia in severe cases

When elements of expressive and receptive dysphasia are present together, the patient is said to have global dysphasia. Global dysphasia results from large lesions and is common in stroke in the territory of the middle cerebral artery.

Differential diagnosis of dysphasia
Parkinson's disease, depressive illness and dementia usually result in reduced verbal fluency and may be confused with expressive dysphasia. On the other hand, patients with receptive dysphasia may be misdiagnosed as having an acute mental confusional state, especially if there are no other focal neurological deficits. The disintegration of language function that occurs in advanced dementia may also be confused for dysphasia.

Treatment and prognosis
Speech and language therapy is the mainstay of dysphasia treatment. It appears to be most effective when therapy is started early and is given for at least the first three months after the disease onset. Patients with severe expressive dysphasia may also benefit from aids that enhance or substitute verbal communication (augmentative and alternative communication). There is a wide range of these aids and they are usually effective if chosen carefully.

The prognosis for recovery from severe dysphasia is generally poor. For example, with the current methods of treatment only approximately 30% of dysphasic stroke patients show significant functional improvement or complete recovery at 3-6 months. The prognosis is improved in patients with right hemisphere dominance. Left-handed subjects tend to become dysphasic regardless of which hemisphere is damaged, and they often recover faster and more completely than dextral individuals. A high level of formal education is also good prognostic factor.

Dysarthria

Dysarthria is a disorder of articulation of speech. Dysarthric speech is slurred, slow and imprecise. It is often monotonous and dysprosodic. However, the speech is usually intelligible except in severe cases. The intelligibility of dysarthric speech is often affected by other factors, such as fatigue, drowsiness, ill-fitting dentures, mouth ulcers, etc. In routine clinical practice the presence of dysarthria and its severity are confirmed by listening to the patient during spontaneous speech or while reading a short text, or repeating words or sentences at the examiner's request.

Different therapeutic strategies are used to improve the intelligibility of the speech of dysarthric patients. These include voice and prosody training, and exercises to strengthen and improve the coordination of the orofacial musculature. In some cases the use of prostheses, e.g. palatal lift to compensate for hypernasal speech, may improve speech clarity. Various communication aids are also useful in severe cases.

Ideomotor and ideational apraxia

The hallmark of limb apraxia is the patient's inability to complete a learnt motor task successfully. This may be due to difficulties in planning the functional activity (ideational apraxia), or initiating or executing the different components of a task in the correct sequence (ideomotor apraxia).

Diagnosis

The diagnosis of apraxia is frequently missed. Normally, patients do not report their difficulties with the execution of learnt motor skills. In addition, the frequent coexistence of apraxia with dysphasia hampers the detailed assessment of this condition.

Traditionally, screening for apraxia involves asking the patient to carry out a learnt motor act on command, to imitate gestures and to demonstrate the use of common tools and objects. However, there is often a poor correlation between the patient's performance on the pantomimed use of tools and objects and their actual ability to use the same tools and objects in real-life situations. Therefore, the diagnosis of apraxia and the assessment of its severity are best evaluated by observing the patient's performance when carrying out activities of daily living. Particular attention should be paid to the patient's performance of the different constituent parts of the task and the order in which they are performed.

Treatment

The impact of limb apraxia on the patient's functional abilities is often considerable. The presence of severe limb apraxia correlates with high levels of dependency in activities of daily living. In addition, it may limit the ability of the individual to use alternative strategies to compensate for motor impairments. It often also interferes with the successful acquisition of new motor skills during rehabilitation.

To date, there are no universally accepted and successful treatment methods for apraxia. A frequently used method is a reiterative, problem-solving educational process that is underpinned by repeated practice of the deficient motor skill. However, treatment of one apraxic error type does not usually generalise to the improvement for other types of apraxic errors.

Another method is 'strategy training'. This treatment approach is based on the selection of specific functional goals for the individual patient. The interventions are then tailored to address these goals while taking account of the patient's level of functional disability. A hierarchical method of instructions, assistance and feedback are used. Initially, the patient may be asked verbally to carry out the task. If he is unsuccessful, then the therapist gives verbal and non-verbal cues. When the patient fails again to accomplish the task, the therapist proceeds, in this order, to assist through the gestures, then by demonstrating the task and finally by giving 'hands on' assistance. Assistance is gradually withdrawn as the patient's functional abilities increase.

Unilateral hemispatial sensory neglect

Unilateral hemispatial sensory neglect (UHN) is probably the most common and clinically most important cognitive impairment in patients with parietal lobe lesions. For example, it has been estimated that 20 to 90% of patients with non-dominant hemisphere stroke have unilateral hemispatial sensory neglect. It is not difficult to appreciate the impact of severe and persistent UHN on the subject's functional abilities and the potential for social participation. UHN causes difficulties with safe mobility, the performance of activities of daily living, reading and writing, leisure activities and employment. Furthermore, patients with UHN often do not have insight into their difficulties and fail to appreciate the need to engage in rehabilitative interventions.

Clinical features

UHN is frequently associated with hemiplegia. Although peripheral spinothalamic and proprioceptive sensation is usually intact, a visual field defect (usually hemianopia) is often present.

A patient with severe UHN is unaware of events on the affected hemispace. He does not respond to sounds arising in the neglected hemispace or acknowledge the presence of people on that side. The hemiplegic arm often dangles limply by the side of the bed or chair. In addition, when the paralysed leg is caught under the wheelchair, the patient does not show any awareness of this or concern about the potential harm that this may cause. The patient's head is usually turned away from the neglected space. In addition, the patient has no insight into the impairments or their functional consequences, and does not attempt to compensate for his difficulties. This distinguishes UHN from hemianopia.

Differential diagnosis

UHN is often confused with homonymous hemianopia. Although both of these impairments may be present in the same patient, it is important to distinguish between the two. This distinction provides valuable prognostic information on the potential for functional recovery and is also useful for planning the therapeutic interventions. The main features that differentiate UHN from hemianopia are summarised in table 2.2.

Table 2.2
The main features that differentiate hemianopia from unilateral hemispatial neglect (UHN):

Clinical symptom or sign	Hemianopia	UHN
Insight into disability	Intact	Poor
Compensatory head movements	Present	Absent
Spontaneous searching eye movements	Present	Absent or weak
Observation during activities of daily living	No neglect behaviour	Evidence of neglect behaviour
Use of compensatory strategies during functional tasks	Yes	No

Numerous tests are used for the diagnosis of UHN. Observation of the patient's spontaneous behaviour and his response to external stimuli often provide sufficient evidence of the presence or absence of UHN. Further evidence may be obtained from the patient's performance on bedside tests. The line bisection test and the star cancellation tests are reliable and easy to administer and interpret.

The line bisection test is the simplest of these tests. The patient is asked to mark the middle of a single 28 cm long horizontal line drawn on A4 paper. The paper is placed in front of the patient so that it corresponds to the middle of his body. The test result is scored by measuring the deviation of the patient's mark from the true middle point of the line.

In the star cancellation test, the patient is asked to cross out the small stars on a drawing consisting 52 large stars and letters of the English alphabet that are randomly positioned among 54 small stars (27 on each half of the page). UHN is diagnosed when the patient fails to cross out all or most of the small stars in the relevant half of the page. If targets are missed on both sides, it is likely the patient has a deficit of generalised attention, rather than lateralised UHN. An example of the performance of a patient with left UHN on the star cancellation test is shown in figure 2.1.

Figure 2.1
Evidence of left UHN on the star cancellation test. Note that the size of the image is reduced

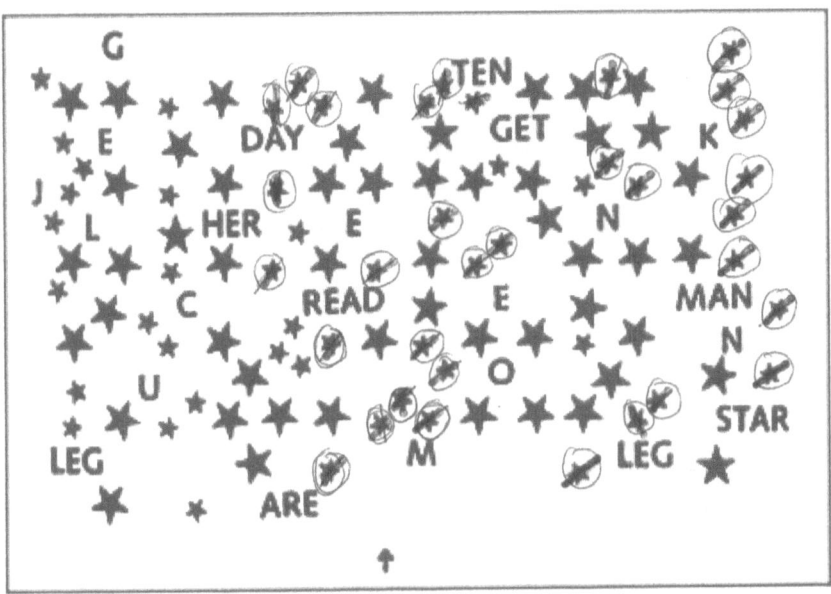

Treatment

Spontaneous recovery occurs in most cases of mild to moderately severe UHN. At present there are no therapeutic interventions that have been conclusively shown to ameliorate the deficits caused by persistent UHN, or to significantly enhance the patient's ability to compensate for them and improve their effects on the patient's normal functional activities. Generally, four therapeutic strategies are used in the rehabilitation of patients with UHN.

1. Methods that attempt to compensate for the symptoms of UHN:
These methods are known as impairment training or transfer of training. They are based on the use of visual, tactile or auditory cues to encourage

the patient to scan and explore the neglected hemispace. These strategies often improve performance in reading and writing tasks, but usually do not generalise with regards to other activities or result in more functional independence.

2. Methods that enhance the patient's awareness of the UHN:
These methods consist of task-specific training. The patient is prompted to direct and maintain his attention to the affected hemispace and is reminded with an alerting device, e.g. a flashing light or bell ringing, when his attention falters. Strategies that improve general attention and arousal and exploit the patient's voluntary attentional mechanisms (such as feedback) also tend to reduce UHN.

3. Methods that orientate the neglected hemispace to the patient's reference frame:
These include the use of eyepatches to cover the visual field ipsilateral to the brain lesion and the use of Fresnel prisms (which can be orientated to displace the retinal image to the left or right as required).

4. The use of dopamine agonists for the treatment of UHN:
It has been claimed that dopamine agonists promote recovery from UHN due to a specific effect on the neural circuits concerned with the exploration of space. However, a non-specific arousal or a motivational effect are also possible. Bromocriptine in a dose of 15 mg daily for 3-4 weeks was reported to have improved the symptoms of chronic UHN. However, the reported beneficial effect of these drugs has not yet been evaluated in large-scale randomised controlled trials.

Impairments of visual function

The nature of visual disturbances depends largely on the site and size of the brain lesion. Optic nerve lesions cause blindness or scotomas. Partial visual field loss is due to damage to the optic tract or corona radiata. By contrast, involvement of the occipital cortex or the parieto-occipital junction usually causes disturbances of visual perception, while patients with brain stem lesions often have double vision.

The typical visual field loss is a homonymous hemianopia or a homonymous quadrantanopia. The patient usually has insight into the visual deficit and often reports difficulties with reading and/or partial blindness. Hemianopia should not be confused with unilateral hemispatial neglect, although the two may coexist. As mentioned in Chapter 1, homonymous hemianopia can be easily confirmed on the bedside assessment of the visual fields with the confrontation method, but sometimes a formal assessment with perimetry may be necessary.

Rarely, patients with occipital lobe stroke and intact eyesight may develop prosopagnosia, colour agnosia or visual object agnosia. The agnosia is related only to the visual modality, and face and object recognition are possible through other sensory modalities, i.e. smell, touch and sound.

There is no curative treatment for prosopagnosia, colour agnosia or visual object agnosia. However, strategies based on the use of the auditory and tactile sensory modalities to compensate for the effects of these impairments are usually effective.

Several methods of treatment for visual field loss, either individually or in combination, may be used. These include visual restitution training with or without attentional cueing, compensatory visual field scanning, manipulation of light conditions and the use of optical devices, such as prisms that relocate the image to the intact area of the visual field. Occlusion of one eye (with an eyepatch or a covered spectacle lens) is often sufficient for the successful management of diplopia, but surgery may be required in chronic, severe cases.

Cognitive impairment

Cognitive impairment is a common consequence of neurodegenerative and cerebrovascular disease. The severity of cognitive impairment may range from mild disturbances of memory to overt dementia. Impairment of memory is usually the earliest and most frequently reported symptom. As the disease progresses, patients develop symptoms that suggest further intellectual deterioration and changes in behaviour and personality. These features are common to all dementias irrespective of the underlying cause.

However, the mode of onset, the clinical course and the presence and nature of focal neurological signs all help to distinguish the various types of dementia.

For example, in contrast to Alzheimer's disease, which starts insidiously and progresses slowly, the onset of vascular dementia is acute and its course is stepwise. The patient usually presents with a focal neurological deficit and symptoms of mental confusion and cognitive impairment. A variable degree of recovery follows and the patient's cognitive state improves slightly or remains stable until the next vascular event. In addition, vascular dementia is usually characterised by less severe memory impairment and more pronounced difficulties with mental concentration than Alzheimer's disease. Typically, the patient has reduced verbal fluency, reduced reaction time, apathy and perseveration.

The physical examination may confirm the presence of hemiparesis or other focal neurological signs that are consistent with brain damage in a vascular territory. Visuospatial deficits are common. In addition, evidence of long-standing hypertension or other risk factors for stroke are often present. The diagnosis may be confirmed with CT or MRI head scans. Typically, these investigations demonstrate the presence of multiple lacunar infarcts (see Chapter 4) in the basal ganglia, internal capsule and centrum semiovale, and widespread white matter changes.

Early dementia may also be confused with depressive illness. However, a carefully taken history and physical examination usually reveal that the underlying problem in patients with primary depression is that of psychomotor retardation, rather than true cognitive impairment. Confirmation to diagnose dementia can be made with psychometric tests, such as the Weschler Adult Intelligence Scale (WAIS).

Treatment
Management of the stroke risk factors and the use of antithrombotic therapy is the mainstay of management in vascular dementia. Three acetylcholinesterase inhibitors (donepezil, rivastigmine and galantamine) have been shown to improve the symptoms of dementia, or to reduce

the rate of cognitive decline in patients with mild or moderately severe Alzheimer's disease. However, their role in the management of vascular dementia is not fully clear at present.

Cognitive rehabilitation may help patients in the early stages of dementia, but it is usually ineffective with advanced disease. The importance of the provision for practical and emotional support to the patients, their families and carers cannot be overemphasised. With adequate social support, including the provision of respite care, most patients with mild or moderately severe vascular dementia are capable of living in the community. However, institutional care is often necessary in the later stages of the disease.

Motor system disorders

Muscle weakness due to neurological disease often leads to a wide range of disabilities. Involvement of facial muscles often causes dysarthria and dysphagia. Weakness of the upper limb may render the hand functionally useless. Patients are usually unable to maintain an independent sitting balance due to weakness of trunk muscles and postural instability. The ability to walk is often lost or severely reduced in cases of paraplegia and tetraplegia.

Assessment

The evaluation of the motor function should include assessment of the muscle strength (e.g. with the MRC scale), muscle tone, and static and dynamic balance.

Assessment of the patient's static and dynamic sitting balance is important because good sitting balance is an essential prerequisite for being able to transfer from one place to another, to stand or to walk. It is usually sufficient to assess the sitting balance by carefully observing the patient during unsupported sitting and during activities that cause perturbation of balance, e.g. raising the unaffected arm, throwing an object or reaching for objects that are placed beyond the arm's length. Similarly, assessment of the standing balance can be made by the clinical observation of postural sway and the symmetry of the distribution of body weight on both legs during standing.

Management

There is no specific treatment that reverses muscle paralysis. Natural recovery of motor function occurs in the vast majority of patients with non-progressive disease, but the extent of improvement and the speed with which it occurs vary widely between individuals. The aim of management is to prevent the complications of muscle paralysis, to enhance the biological recovery and to help the patient learn new strategies to compensate for the motor disability. The development of muscle contractures, shoulder subluxation and other injuries are common but preventable complications in patients with motor weakness.

The prevention and prompt treatment of these complications is, therefore, of paramount importance. Meticulous attention should be paid to the correct positioning of the patient while lying in bed, rolling over in bed and during transfers from bed to chair, and during sitting and standing. The optimal posture is that the shoulder on the hemiplegic side is maintained in a protracted, i.e. a forward, position. The arm is slightly externally rotated and extended at the elbow and wrist. The hip should also be protracted but internally rotated. When the patient is lying in bed, the same posture should be adopted and, in addition, the knee on the hemiplegic side should also be slightly flexed. The same principles should be followed when bridging is attempted, e.g. in order to use a bedpan. (Bridging is lifting the pelvis off the bed while lying prone with the hips and knees flexed.)

The cornerstone of the management of patients with motor weakness is physical therapy. The frequency and duration of physiotherapy sessions appear to correlate with the degree motor functional recovery. Apart from conventional physiotherapy, several other therapeutic modalities have been introduced for the treatment of motor weakness in recent years. These include constraint-induced therapy, treadmill training, biofeedback, functional electrical stimulation and the use of robotic devices.

Course and prognosis

Motor recovery usually follows a predictable pattern. It usually starts in the proximal muscles groups. Distal muscles, especially muscles of the upper limb, tend to recover last and their recovery is usually limited. Most of the functional recovery occurs in the first three months after the onset of non-progressive neurological diseases, such as stroke.

Muscle spasticity

Muscle spasticity is an important cause of severe locomotor disability in patients with the upper motor neuron syndrome. Spastic dystonia, flexor and extensor muscle spasms and associated limb reactions are also common in patients with spasticity. All of these phenomena or any combination may occur in the same patient.

Spasticity frequently results in impairment of voluntary movements, interferes with safe ambulation, causes muscle pain and predisposes to fixed muscle contractures. However, it should also be remembered that spasticity is often functionally useful. It is invaluable for the maintenance of trunk posture, weight bearing on the weak lower limb and for ambulation. Other possible beneficial effects include the prevention of deep vein thrombosis in the paretic limb and the maintenance of muscle mass and bone density. Therefore, the management of patients with spasticity should be based on a careful neurological examination and a detailed functional evaluation.

The management of spasticity

The aim of management is to assess the severity of spasticity, to establish the extent of the functional disability due to the increased muscle tone, to clearly define the desired outcomes of treatment, to choose the most appropriate therapeutic interventions and to select the methods to monitor the effects of treatment.

The indications for treatment

A common indication for treatment of muscle spasticity is to alleviate distressing symptoms, such as painful spasms. In some cases, the aim is to improve motor function or to prevent or reduce the complications of muscle hypertonia including fixed contractures and joint dislocations. In patients with severe spasticity of the lower limb muscles, the hypertonia often prevents comfortable and safe sitting in a chair or positioning in bed. Treatment of spasticity of the ankle plantar flexors is indicated in cases of dynamic foot equinus that result in difficulties with safe and energy efficient walking, and spasticity that prevents the effective use of an ankle-foot orthosis. Treatment may also be considered when sustained ankle clonus interferes with ambulation by preventing the correct heel contact with the ground, or when it causes difficulties with foot placement on the footplate of a wheelchair.

Treatment options

Several treatment modalities are used for the relief of muscle spasticity. These are antispasticity drugs, chemical neurolysis, botulinum toxin injections, physiotherapy, splinting and the use of plaster casts, and surgery. The selection of the treatment modality depends on whether the spasticity is localised or generalised, what the treatment goals are, the available resources and the clinician's expertise. However, as a general rule, the use of different treatment modalities together results in greater symptomatic improvement and better functional outcomes than when only one type of intervention is used.

Many conditions, including urinary tract infections, pressure sores, faecal impaction, ingrown toenails and contractures may aggravate muscle spasticity. These conditions should be routinely looked for in patients with spasticity and appropriately managed when present.

Oral antispasticity drugs are useful in patients with generalised spasticity. The major oral antispasticity drugs are baclofen, benzodiazepines, dantrolene and tizanidine. These drugs reduce muscle tone by different mechanisms and may be used in combination.

Treatment with baclofen should be started with a small dose (e.g. 5 mg three times per day). The dose is then titrated up over 2-3 weeks until the desired effect on spasticity is obtained. In most patients this can be achieved with a total daily dose of 60 mg. Discontinuation of treatment with baclofen should be gradual and at least over 2 weeks. The sudden withdrawal of this drug after prolonged use may precipitate serious complications including epileptic seizures and hallucinations.

Diazepam is a very potent antispasticity agent but doses of up to 60 mg/day may be required before a good clinical effect can be achieved. The use of the benzodiazepines for the treatment of spasticity is limited by their adverse effects, which include sedation, amnesia and mental confusion. In addition, the chronic use of the benzodiazepines in high doses is associated with the risk of drug dependence and depression. Paradoxically, the long-term use of diazepam may increase muscle spasticity, precipitate an anxiety state, aggression and insomnia.

Dantrolene is also an effective antispasticity drug with an adverse effect profile similar to that of baclofen. In addition, very rarely it can cause hepatic failure. The incidence of the hepatic adverse effects correlates with the dose of dantrolene and the duration of treatment. They seldom occur in patients receiving less than 400 mg/day (which is the maximum recommended dose) or in the first 2 months of treatment. It is recommended that liver function is monitored at regular intervals after the commencement of treatment.

Tizanidine has an antispasticity effect similar to that of baclofen and diazepam. It is claimed that tizanidine has the additional advantage of reducing muscle tone without causing muscle weakness, and that it is particularly effective in younger patients and in those with very severe spasticity, especially when pain in the spastic muscle is a prominent feature. In most cases the optimal dose of tizanidine is 16 mg/day. Treatment is usually started with a small dose, e.g. 2 mg daily. The dose is then increased gradually every third day until the desired effect on muscle tone is obtained. The main adverse effects of this drug are dose-dependent and include sedation, bradycardia and hypotension.

Large doses of oral antispasticity drugs often produce generalised muscle weakness. This is a major drawback because the reduction of muscle strength may increase the functional disability, especially when trunk and other postural muscles are affected. Sometimes these drugs reduce muscle strength in the unaffected extremities without significantly reducing the spasticity or improving function of the spastic limbs. Furthermore, the value of oral antispasticity drugs usually diminishes with prolonged use. Tolerance frequently develops after a few months of treatment, and incremental increases in dosage are often required to maintain the same clinical response. This usually increases the incidence and severity of the dose-dependent adverse effects of these drugs.

Botulinum toxin injections and the destruction of peripheral nerves with local injections of phenol or alcohol (chemical neurolysis) are effective methods of treatment of localised muscle hypertonia and are often combined with physiotherapy and the use of splints and plaster casts. Surgery is indicated when severe muscle contractures cause functional disability.

Limb and trunk ataxia

Ataxia may result from direct damage to the cerebellum (cerebellar ataxia) or from impairment or loss of proprioception (sensory ataxia).

Mild limb ataxia is usually asymptomatic and is detected on clinical examination with the finger–nose test and the heel–shin test. As a rule it has no effect on motor function. In moderately severe ataxia, the motor activity is carried out in a clumsy, uncoordinated way. The trajectory of the limb movement is inaccurate, but the intended motor task is frequently accomplished, albeit with difficulty. By contrast, in severe ataxia the limb frequently misses the target and the patient is unable to use his limb effectively. Trunk ataxia causes difficulties with sitting unsupported and walking.

Ataxia may interfere with the patient's mobility and activities of daily living, including feeding, and personal care. Different methods are used for the management of ataxia. The main therapeutic intervention consists of stabilisation of the proximal limb segment combined with balance training and visual feedback. Other treatment strategies are less effective and include the use of wrist weights to reduce upper limb excursion (in order to control the range and direction of movement) and the prescription of drugs, such as isoniazid (900-1200 mg/day), primidone (250-750 mg/day) and propranolol (40-120 mg/day).

Bladder and bowel dysfunction

Bladder and bowel dysfunction in neurological patients can be either due to the neurological disorder itself or a coincidental condition, such as prostatic hypertrophy or stress incontinence. The main bladder disorders associated with neurological disease are detrusor hyperreflexia, detrusor-sphincter dyssynergia and detrusor hyperreflexia (for details see section 3.10 of the previous chapter).

Assessment

A carefully taken micturitional history followed by abdominal and rectal examination is the cornerstone of diagnosis of bladder dysfunction.

Irritative symptoms, such as frequency, urgency and nocturia, are characteristic of detrusor-sphincter dyssynergia and detrusor hyperreflexia/ instability. However, the combination of these symptoms with dysuria usually indicates the presence of an uncomplicated urinary tract infection (UTI). The symptoms of bladder neck obstruction are voiding difficulty, urinary hesitancy and weak stream of urine. Leakage of urine when coughing or sneezing is a sign of stress incontinence.

Initial screening of patients with bladder dysfunction should include urine microscopy and culture. In patients with obstructive urinary symptoms, a bladder ultrasound scan is a useful non-invasive method for demonstrating the cause (e.g. a large prostate) and for measuring the post-voiding residual volume. Intravenous urography may be necessary to demonstrate the presence or confirm the absence of dilatation of the ureters and the pelvicalyceal renal system. Evaluation of the renal function and the measurement of serum electrolytes are also an essential part of the patient's initial screening and subsequent monitoring. Specialist investigations, such as video urodynamic studies, are sometimes required to distinguish between the different types of urinary incontinence.

Treatment

There are two main goals of treatment of neurogenic bladder dysfunction, irrespective of the underlying cause or the mechanism of incontinence. The first aim is to protect renal function and the second is to promote continence.

The main measures that help to preserve renal function are the prevention and prompt treatment of UTI and ureteric reflux. Intermittent self-catheterisation (at least four times a day) is a useful management strategy in patients with neurogenic bladder dysfunction, especially in the presence of chronic or recurrent urinary tract infections. Sphincterotomy is indicated for detrusor-sphincter dyssynergia in order to safeguard against ureteric reflux and renal damage.

Promotion of urinary continence is achievable with bladder training (scheduled voiding) in approximately 50% of patients. The patient is asked to urinate initially every two hours with progressive lengthening of the periods between voiding until continence is re-established. When these measures fail, continence may be achieved by the use of condom (penile sheath) drainage, incontinence pads, a dribble pouch or other similar devices. Long-term catheterisation should be considered a last resort in the management of urinary incontinence. Silicon catheters are preferable to latex catheters and can be left in situ for 6-8 weeks.

Drug treatment of urinary incontinence should also be considered. Antimuscarinic drugs, such as oxybutynin and tolterodine, inhibit the activity of the detrusor muscle and are frequently used in the treatment of detrusor hyperreflexia and detrusor instability. Oxybutynin is usually started in a dose of 2.5 mg once a day. The dose is then titrated up in increments of 2.5 mg every 3-4 days until the patient is continent, or to a maximum dose of 5 mg three times a day. The slow release version of oxybutynin is as effective and is better tolerated than the standard preparation. Tolterodine 2 mg twice a day is an alternative to oxybutynin.

Bowel dysfunction
The neurological causes of faecal incontinence are frontal lobe, pyramidal tract, spinal cord and sacral root lesions. Non-neurological causes include severe constipation resulting in faecal impaction and overflow of soft stools, laxative abuse, immobility (especially if combined with severe communication difficulties due to dysphasia or dysarthria), cognitive impairment, and coincidental surgical and obstetric disorders that compromise the integrity of the anal sphincter, such as rectal or vaginal prolapse.

Assessment

The evaluation of a faecally incontinent patient should include assessment of the severity of the incontinence and a diagnostic workup of its underlying cause. The severity of faecal incontinence can be established from the history and physical examination. Severe faecal incontinence is characterised by frequent loss of bowel control irrespective of the consistency of the stools. By contrast, in cases of mild incontinence the patients soil their underpants with small amounts of loose or semi-formed stools. Mild incontinence should not be confused with soiling due to prolapsed haemorroids, an anal fistula or vaginal discharge.

A carefully taken history and clinical examination are often sufficient to elucidate the cause of faecal incontinence. Inspection of the perineum may confirm the presence of a rectal or vaginal prolapse or scarring from a previous episiotomy. An absent anocutaneous reflex suggests disruption of the sacral reflex arc due to a neuropathy or a cauda equina lesion. A lax anal sphincter on rectal examination would suggest incompetence of the anal sphincter, and the presence of a large amount of hard faeces in the rectum is diagnostic of faecal impaction. Specialist investigations, such as anal manometry, endoanal ultrasound, anorectal electromyography and nerve conduction studies of the pudendal nerve may be needed, especially if surgical treatment is being considered.

Management

Treatment of faecal incontinence should aim to correct the underlying cause of incontinence whenever possible. Faecal impaction and overflow incontinence should be treated with regular phosphate or hypertonic enemas. In some cases manual evacuation of the rectum may be required. Adequate hydration and a high fibre diet should be encouraged in order to prevent recurrence.

Patients with faecal incontinence due to neurogenic causes may benefit from treatment with loperamide, which increases anal pressures. Regular toileting at a specified time every day may also help to re-establish continence. This intervention is most effective when the bowel training is tailored to mimic the patient's previous bowel habit. When medical management fails, different surgical procedures may be used for the treatment of faecal incontinence. These include external anal sphincter repair, mechanical tightening of the anus, e.g. with a silastic ring, implantation of an artificial anal sphincter and even colostomy. Sometimes the only realistic management option is the use of continence pads and other incontinence aids.

Dysphagia

Normal swallowing depends on the anatomical and functional integrity of numerous neural structures and extensive pathways in the central and peripheral nervous systems. Lesions in the cerebral cortex, basal ganglia, brain stem, cerebellum or peripheral nerves may interrupt these pathways. Muscle disease may also cause swallowing difficulties. This explains the high incidence of dysphagia in neurological patients.

Several drugs may also precipitate or aggravate swallowing difficulties. The mechanisms implicated in this are diverse and include depression of the level of consciousness (sedatives and hypnotics), interference with the oropharyngeal phase of swallowing (e.g. neuroleptic agents), or poor preparation of the food bolus due to xerostomia (dry mouth) caused by anticholinergic drugs.

The clinical manifestations of dysphagia

Patients with mild or moderately severe dysphagia may not be aware of their swallowing difficulties. These patients usually avoid certain foods that they find difficult to chew or swallow. Weight loss may be an early feature in some cases. Excessive flow and drooling of saliva (sialorrhoea) occurs in dysphagic patients when they are sitting up, and pulmonary aspiration of saliva is common in the recumbent position, especially during sleep. Pain on swallowing (odynophagia) is not a symptom of neurogenic dysphagia and suggests a diagnosis of oesophagitis, usually secondary to candida infections. Nasal regurgitation of fluids occurs when palatal weakness is present.

Assessment

Assessment of swallowing function should start with a careful examination of the oral cavity. Some causes of dysphagia, such as mouth ulcers, oral thrush, xerostomia and deviation of the soft palate are readily visible on inspection of the patient's mouth. Neurological examination may confirm the presence of bulbar or pseudobulbar palsy, Bell's palsy or weakness of the orobuccal muscles on the hemiplegic side.

The presence of dysphagia and its severity can then be assessed at the bedside by observing the patient during 'trial swallows'. Coughing, spluttering or choking while eating are obvious signs of dysphagia. Change in the pattern of breathing or change in voice quality may also occur. Some patients attempt to compensate for their swallowing difficulties by taking small, frequent drinks during the meal in order to 'wash down' the food bolus. Inspection of the oral cavity usually reveals pooling of secretions or food residue in the mouth.

Video fluoroscopy is considered the gold standard for the evaluation of dysphagia. It permits the observation of the oral preparatory phase, the reflex initiation of swallowing and the pharyngeal transit of the food bolus. However, it is not suitable for repeated assessments because of the undesirability of frequent exposure to radiation and the cost of the procedure.

Differential diagnosis

Neurogenic dysphagia should be differentiated from dysphagia due to obstructive lesions and dysphagia due to other non-neurological causes. Obstructive lesions of the oesophagus usually cause slowly progressive dysphagia. Typically, the patient reports difficulties with swallowing solid food in the early stages. By contrast, patients with neurogenic dysphagia usually find fluids more difficult to swallow than solids. This is probably because a solid (and more cohesive) food bolus is more likely to result in adequate pharyngeal stimulation and thus triggers a swallow reflex.

Management

Dysphagia is a potential cause of pulmonary aspiration, dehydration, reduced calorie intake and malnutrition. The aim of management is to prevent these complications, to maintain adequate food and fluid intake and to correct nutritional deficiencies when present.

Oral feeding has important social and psychological significance to patients and their families and should be continued whenever possible. In some patients, oral intake is often not adequate even in the absence of significant swallowing difficulties. This may be due to excessive fatigue or cognitive impairment. In these patients, oral food intake may be supplemented with gastrostomy tube feeding. It is preferable that such supplements are given at night. Withholding morning gastrostomy feeds usually stimulates the patient's appetite.

Review of the patient's medication
Sedatives, hypnotic drugs and tranquillisers often reduce the patient's level of arousal and render swallowing unsafe. They should not be used whenever possible. Anticholinergic drugs, e.g. hyoscine patches, are sometimes prescribed for dysphagic patients with excessive drooling of saliva. Drooling of saliva in these patients is due to difficulties with swallowing and not because of its excessive production. Consequently, these drugs should be avoided as they can aggravate dysphagia by increasing the viscosity of oral secretions. Similarly, antihistamines and tricyclic antidepressants also increase the viscosity of oral secretions. Viscid oral secretions interfere with bolus preparation and predispose to the formation of a mucous plug. Dehydration, e.g. due to the use of diuretics, may also have a similar effect. The antiemetics prochlorperazine and metoclopramide may occasionally cause orofacial dyskinesia, and this could result in dysphagia or aggravate pre-existing swallowing difficulties.

Dietary modification
Maintenance of hydration and nutrition can be achieved safely in most patients with neurogenic dysphagia with dietary modification. Simple, but effective, measures include avoidance of dry and sticky food and eating food with uniform consistency. The use of starch-based fluid thickeners, e.g. Thick and Easy™ and Vitaquick®, is also an important management strategy. Tube feeding is usually required in only a minority of patients.

Tube feeding
The direct delivery of nutrients into the stomach (or rarely into the jejunum) via a feeding tube is frequently used as the sole method of nutritional

support for severely dysphagic patients who are at risk of pulmonary aspiration, if fed orally.

The use of a gastrostomy tube is preferred to nasoesophageal intubation, especially when dysphagia is expected to be present for more than a few days. Nasogastric tube (NGT) feeding is usually poorly tolerated and may make the patient irritable or even agitated. Removal of the tube by patients is common and the volume of feeds delivered in this way is usually not adequate. Frequently, only half the required daily nutritional intake can be delivered using an NGT. Prolonged NGT feeding is not desirable. It may result in numerous complications including nasopharyngitis, oesophagitis, oesophageal strictures, epistaxis, pneumothorax and nasopharyngeal oedema with associated otitis media. If dysphagia is expected to continue for more than 3-4 weeks, the option of percutaneous endoscopic gastrostomy (PEG) tube feeding should be considered.

Swallowing therapy

A range of remedial therapies and training in the use of compensatory strategies may be helpful in the treatment of neurogenic dysphagia. These include exercises to strengthen the orofacial musculature, methods to improve poor laryngeal elevation and laryngeal closure during swallowing, and techniques to stimulate the swallow reflex.

The surgical treatment of neurogenic dysphagia

Cricopharyngeal myotomy has been shown to be an effective method of treatment of dysphagia in a number of neurological disorders including stroke, muscular dystrophy and a significant proportion of patients with motor neurone disease. However, careful selection of patients for this procedure is essential and two conditions must be satisfied. Firstly, failure of relaxation of the pharyngeal sphincter must be demonstrated on video fluoroscopy. Secondly, the oral phase of swallowing i.e. lip seal, voluntary initiation of swallowing and the propulsive action of the tongue, must also be preserved. Poor tongue movements is a contraindication to cricopharyngeal myotomy. Patients with absent pharyngeal peristalsis or delayed triggering of the swallow reflex by 10 seconds or more are also unlikely to benefit from this treatment.

Disturbances of mood and emotions

Major and minor mood disorders are common in patients with neurological disease who have no history of mental illness. Anxiety often coexists with depression. Irritability, impulsivity and emotional lability may also occur. The mechanisms of depression in these patients are not entirely clear. The grievance for the functional loss, altered family and social roles and perceived low self-worth as a result of disability may be important factors in the aetiopathogenesis. Anxiety is often attributed to fear of death or worries about disability, fear of abandonment by a spouse, or feeling of helplessness. Sometimes it is a plea by the patient for attention.

Assessment

A clinical diagnosis of depression is made if the patient has a combination of easily recognisable symptoms, such as abnormally low mood, anhedonia, i.e. abnormal loss in pleasure, morbid thoughts of death or suicide, inappropriate guilt and self-reproach, and behavioural disturbances, e.g. agitation or retardation. However, the classical symptoms of depression may be absent. Depression should be suspected in cases of poor, delayed or erratic functional recovery; in the persistence of disability that is disproportionate to the severity of the neurological deficit; unexplained functional deterioration after an initial good improvement; and emotional lability, i.e. pathological laughing and crying, in the absence of pseudobulbar palsy.

Treatment

Although psychotherapy is usually effective in mild depression, drug treatment is almost always necessary in cases of severe or moderately severe depression. As a rule, the selective serotonin reuptake inhibitors are better tolerated than tricyclic antidepressants, but the latter tend to be more effective. The beneficial effect of antidepressant drugs is usually observed 2-3 weeks after the start of therapy. However, if the patient's symptoms persist after 4-6 weeks of treatment with the appropriate drug dose, change of the antidepressant medication should be considered. It is recommended that the antidepressant treatment is continued for at least 6 months after the complete recovery from depression. Early withdrawal of treatment may precipitate a relapse of symptoms. The withdrawal of antidepressant drugs should be gradual over several weeks. Abrupt cessation of treatment should be avoided, except when serious adverse effects develop.

CHAPTER 3

DISORDERS OF CONSCIOUSNESS

Consciousness is defined as a combination of arousal (wakefulness/alertness or sleep-wake cycles) and awareness of self and of the surrounding environment. It is maintained by the activity of the cerebral cortex, thalamus, and reticular formation and their neuronal connections. The disturbances of consciousness result from damage to these structures and range in severity from coma, to the vegetative state and minimally conscious state.

The bedside assessment of the level of consciousness is usually made with various clinical scales. The modified Glasgow Coma Scale (GCS) is probably the best known and most widely used method to assess the level of consciousness and for monitoring its improvement (or deterioration) over time. The GCS consists of three subscales, namely eye opening, verbal response and motor response. The items of each subscale and their scores are shown in the table 3.1 below.

Table 3.1
The Glasgow Coma Scale:

Subscale	Item	score
Eye opening	No eye opening	1
	Eyes open in response to painful stimuli	2
	Eyes open in response to voice	3
	Eyes open spontaneously	4

Verbal response	No verbal response	1
	Patient makes incomprehensible sounds	2
	Patient says inappropriate words	3
	Patient able to speak but confused	4
	Patient able to converse normally	5
Motor response	No movements	1
	Limb extension to pain	2
	Limb flexion to pain	3
	Limb withdrawal to pain	4
	Patient localises pain	5
	Obeys commands	6

The maximum summated GCS score is 15 and means that the subject is fully awake. The lowest possible score is 3. Severe loss of consciousness is defined as a GCS score of 8 or less. A score of 9-12 and 13-14 respectively indicate moderately severe or mild impairment of consciousness.

Coma

When both components of consciousness, i.e. alertness and awareness, are lost, the patient is said to be in a coma. There is no spontaneous eye opening or voluntary movements and no response to commands. Reflex movements may be present. The score of 10 or less on the Glasgow Coma Scale is usually used as an indication of coma.

Traumatic brain injury, stroke, anoxia, poisoning, epilepsy, CNS infections, metabolic disorders, e.g. hypoglycaemia, hepatic or renal encephalopathy, are the most common causes of coma. In tropical countries, cerebral malaria is an important cause of coma.

The persistent and permanent vegetative state

The vegetative state (also called the Unresponsive Wakefulness Syndrome – UWS) is characterised by complete loss of awareness of self and of the surrounding environment while the vegetative functions (spontaneous breathing, heartbeat and sleep-wake cycles) are preserved. The patient opens and closes his eyes spontaneously, but he does not respond to commands or sensory stimuli and does not make purposeful movements.

The term 'persistent vegetative state' is generally used if the condition lasts more than one month. If the symptoms last 12 months or more in a patient with traumatic brain injury or 3 months or more if the coma is due to a non-traumatic cause, the term permanent vegetative state (PVS) is used.

PVS is usually preceded by coma in cases of traumatic brain injury and anoxic brain damage, but, in rare cases, it can develop without a preceding coma in patients with severe metabolic or neurodegenerative disease.

The minimally conscious state (MCS)

In contrast to PVS, a patient who is minimally conscious has any or all of the following signs: the ability to follow simple commands, verbalise and produce purposeful movements or emotional responses. These behaviours can be either sustained or reproducible. However, the distinction between PVS and MCS is sometimes difficult and various investigations (e.g. functional MRI, studies of cerebral glucose metabolism with positron emission tomography, and EEG) are used to differentiate between these conditions.

Management and prognosis of coma, PVS and MCS

Care of the comatose involves treating the underlying cause and general life support measures. However, when treatment is considered futile a decision about the continuation of the therapeutic interventions needs to be made. Important legal and ethical issues surround the decisions to withdraw life support and other treatments in cases of PVS and MCS. Therefore, in addition to the physician's conclusion of the futility of treatment, compliance with the country's laws, respect for the patient's wishes (e.g. stated in an advanced directive) and his religious beliefs are essential for decision-making in such situations.

The prognosis of coma depends on its cause. Coma due to stroke has the worst prognosis. By contrast, full recovery from coma caused by poisoning is common. Coma is considered irreversible and brain death is diagnosed if the patient (who is not hypothermic or hypotensive, and has not taken sedative or hypnotic drugs) has no spontaneous breathing or muscle activity, no brain stem reflexes and an electrically silent EEG for 6 hours or more.

The prognosis of PVS and MCS is poor. Recovery is very unlikely after 12 months if the condition is caused by traumatic brain injury, or after 3 months if it is due to other causes. However, in the rare event the patient recovers after 2 or 3 years, he is invariably left with severe permanent neurological disability. Young subjects and those with PVS/MCS due to traumatic brain injury appear to have a better prognosis.

Epilepsy

Epilepsy is a neurological disorder characterised by recurrent attacks of loss or alteration of consciousness, convulsive movements, psychic symptoms and abnormal sensations (which occur in various combinations). The disorder is caused by a sudden excessive abnormal electric discharge of a group of cerebral neurons (the epileptogenic focus). The spread of the discharge to the rest of the brain results in a generalised seizure. Epilepsy is the most common neurological disease after stroke. Its prevalence in the general population is approximately 1%. The highest incidence of epilepsy is in childhood and old age.

The cause of epilepsy is often unknown (idiopathic epilepsy), but in some cases it is a complication of an identifiable brain disease or systemic illness (symptomatic epilepsy). In idiopathic epilepsy, a family history is common and genetic factors appear to be important. For example, if an identical twin develops epilepsy, the risk for the other twin is more than 50%. However, a direct link between epilepsy and genetic mutations is rare and is mainly found in the epileptic encephalopathies of infancy and early childhood. There is no structural abnormality in the brain in cases of idiopathic epilepsy.

Epilepsy is classified into generalised and focal. The main types of generalised epilepsy are tonic-clonic (or grand mal) seizures and absence (or petit mal) seizures. There are three types of focal epilepsy: simple partial seizures, complex partial seizures and partial seizures with secondary generalisation. In some patients a certain stimulus, e.g. flashing light or sudden noise, may trigger an epileptic seizure. This is known as reflex epilepsy.

Febrile convulsions

Some children develop convulsions, usually tonic-clonic, when they have high fever. The typical age of occurrence of these febrile convulsions is between 6 months and 5 years, and in most cases they are self-limiting. However, febrile convulsions that are focal, prolonged or recurrent have a less benign prognosis. Approximately 6 to 7% of children with febrile convulsions develop epilepsy in the future.

Clinical features

Generalised tonic-clonic (grand mal) seizures

This is the most common form of epilepsy and accounts for more than 50% of all cases. Its onset is often preceded by prodromal symptoms that start 30 minutes to several hours before the seizure and usually consist of mood, cognitive or behavioural changes. Anxiety, poor concentration and difficulties with short-term memory, and irritability are common. Some patients experience a warning of an impending seizure (aura) in the form of an unusual sensation in the stomach, palpitations, perception of an unpleasant smell or taste, tingling or other symptoms. The aura is followed by sudden loss of consciousness. The patient falls to the ground, and the limb and trunk muscles become rigid. This is the tonic phase. It lasts approximately 20 seconds and is followed by the clonic phase.

The clonic phase is characterised by violent convulsive limb movements and cessation of breathing. The patient becomes cyanotic, often bites his tongue and froth forms in his mouth. Urinary and/or faecal incontinence is common. Once the convulsive movements stop the muscles become limp, the patient starts to breathe quietly and either wakes up or the unconscious state continues into natural sleep that may last for hours. On waking up the patient is often disorientated, exhausted and may complain of a headache but has no memory of the epileptic seizure. Some patients become paralysed for hours or even days after an epileptic seizure (Todd's paralysis). The cause of Todd's paralysis is not clear. It has been speculated that the paralysis results from 'neuronal exhaustion' due to local metabolic changes triggered by the epileptic discharge. An alternative view is that it results from excessive post-ictal neuronal inhibition. Some patients have only either the tonic or the clonic component of the seizure.

Absence (petit mal) seizures

This form of epilepsy starts in childhood and frequently becomes less severe in later life. It is characterised by frequent, very brief periods of interruption in consciousness and subtle stereotyped motor activities, such lip smacking, swallowing, chewing or fluttering of the eyelids. The child pauses in what he is doing and after a few seconds he resumes the activity without being aware of the event. Many such attacks may happen in quick succession. Myoclonic jerks and tonic-clonic seizures may also be present.

Simple partial seizures

Focal seizures result from the presence of a discrete 'epileptogenic focus' in part of the cerebral cortex. The clinical presentation depends on the location of the lesion. Lesions of the frontal cortex result in motor partial seizures. Typically, the symptoms start on one side of the face, one hand or one foot, and then spread to involve the whole side of the body (this is known as Jacksonian epilepsy). In some patients, the head and eyes turn to the side opposite to the lesion. When the focal seizures become repetitive and continue for a long period the condition is called Epilepsia Partialis Continua.

Symptoms due to localisation of the epileptogenic focus in the sensory cortex include tingling sensations, 'pin and needles', feelings of warmth or cold on the side opposite to the focus (simple partial sensory seizures). Visual hallucinations and visual distortions (macropsia or micropsia) occur with lesions of the occipital cortex, while auditory hallucinations are due lesions in the temporal lobe.

Partial seizures with secondary generalisation

All types of partial seizures start with focal symptoms and signs, but sometimes loss of consciousness ensues and the tonic-clonic sequence of grand mal epilepsy develops.

Complex partial seizures
(also known as temporal lobe epilepsy or psychomotor epilepsy)

The epileptogenic focus in complex partial seizures is in the medial temporal lobe, amygdala and hippocampus. In contrast to the other types of partial seizures, this form of focal epilepsy is characterised by a distinctive aura, automatic behaviour and post-ictal confusion and amnesia.

The aura may consist of many symptoms, including hallucinations of smell or taste, strange epigastric sensations, an impression of familiarity with people, situations and surroundings not previously known to the patient (déjà vu) or the opposite experience (jamais vu). Intense fear, aggression or anxiety are also common. Any combination of these symptoms may occur in the same patient.

Unconscious semi-purposeful motor behaviour (automatism) is a characteristic feature of complex partial seizures. It is either simple or very complex. Examples of simple automatic behaviour are chewing, lip smacking, licking, and purposeless movements of the hands or feet. Some patients carry out complex motor acts such as walking, dressing or undressing or even driving a motor car without being aware of their actions. Nor do they remember them on recovery from the seizure.

Juvenile myoclonic epilepsy (JME)
JME, as the name implies, starts in adolescence. It is a combination of tonic-clonic seizures and myoclonus. (Myoclonus is very brief, involuntary jerky movements.) Although JME responds well to treatment with sodium valproate, it seldom remits and treatment is usually required for life.

Generalised convulsive status epilepticus
Generalised convulsive status epilepticus (GCSE) is defined as epileptic seizures that continue without full recovery of consciousness for 30 minutes or more. It is often triggered by the sudden withdrawal of anticonvulsant drugs, anticonvulsant drug toxicity, sepsis or other severe intercurrent illness.

Diagnosis
The diagnosis of idiopathic epilepsy is made after 2 or more unprovoked seizures that occur at least 24 hours apart. (Provoked seizures are seizures that are due to a complication of systemic or brain disease, such as fever, alcohol withdrawal, head trauma, etc.) A reliable diagnosis of epilepsy can

often be made from the account of an eyewitness and the recording of an electroencephalogram (EEG). Other investigations may also be required.

The EEG is useful for confirming the diagnosis of epilepsy and also for the classification of the seizure type. In grand mal seizures, the EEG recording during the attack (ictal EEG) shows characteristic changes for each stage of the seizure activity. Spike discharges appear at the beginning of the seizure (figure 3.1). Then the discharges increase progressively in frequency and amplitude and spread over the whole cortex. These changes correspond to the tonic phase. In the clonic phase, the discharges become intermittent and less frequent before they stop with the end of the clonic phase. In the post-ictal period, the EEG is characterised by generalised slow waves.

Figure 3.1
The typical EEG of tonic-clonic epilepsy

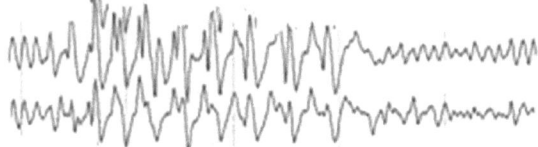

The typical EEG in petit mal (absence) epilepsy consists of three-per-second spike and wave activity in all EEG leads (figure 3.2). However, in some atypical cases the duration of each spike and wave cycle is less than three seconds.

Figure 3.2
The typical EEG of petit mal epilepsy

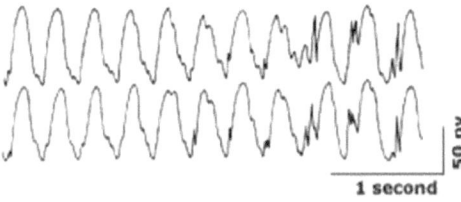

50 pv

1 second

The first standard scalp EEG recording between epileptic seizures (inter-ictal EEG) is normal in one third of epileptic patients who are not taking anticonvulsant medication, and this figure is higher in those on treatment. Some techniques, e.g. flashing lights, deep breathing to induce alkalosis and recording during natural or drug-induced sleep, are often used to improve the diagnostic yield of EEG. When routine and sleep EEG are combined, epilepsy can be confirmed in 80% of patients. Repeated EEG testing also increases the chance of detecting the seizure activity. The simultaneous video and continuous EEG recording (EEG telemetry) is useful in some cases.

Symptomatic epilepsy should be suspected when the disease starts in middle or old age, especially with focal seizures and also when focal neurological signs are present on examination. These cases warrant a further diagnostic workup, including brain imaging.

Differential diagnosis of epilepsy
Misdiagnosis of epilepsy is common. Yet, it is important to make an accurate diagnosis of epilepsy because, in most cases, treatment is needed for many years or even for life. In addition, the diagnosis of epilepsy usually imposes some restrictions on the patient's lifestyle, and has implications for employment and driving a motor vehicle. It is also associated with stigma in some communities.

Syncope and pseudoseizures are the main conditions that mimic epilepsy. Other disorders that may be confused with epilepsy include hypoglycaemia, paroxysmal movement disorders (e.g. dystonia), migraine aura, parasomnias (narcolepsy, cataplexy and, in children, night terrors), panic attacks and paroxysmal vertigo.

Syncope occurs when the systolic blood pressure drops significantly resulting in severe global cerebral ischaemia and transient loss of consciousness. It is caused by simple vasovagal attacks or cardiac disease. A vasovagal syncope (benign, simple faint) is often preceded by dizziness, light-headedness, sweating or nausea. It usually occurs in hot crowded environments; in response to pain, strong emotions or fear; or after prolonged standing. Loss of consciousness is frequently accompanied by tonic or clonic muscle activity, but tongue biting, urinary incontinence or post-ictal confusion are not features of the attack. Patients presenting with syncope due to cardiac disease are usually middle-aged or elderly with a history of heart disease. Ambulatory ECG monitoring and other cardiac investigations are often required for confirmation of the diagnosis.

Pseudoseizures (also called psychogenic non-epileptic seizures) are the most common disorder that may be confused with epilepsy. Although they suggest a personality disorder or mental illness, they may also occur in patients with established epilepsy. Pseudoseizures may resemble tonic-clonic, complex partial or petit mal epilepsy. They are more common in females.

In contrast to epilepsy, pseudoseizures typically occur in the presence of other people and are often triggered by emotional factors. They usually occur in clusters of multiple attacks. The presentation includes focal or generalised movements with or without apparent loss of consciousness. Post-ictal confusion is absent. In addition, other symptoms, e.g. bizarre behaviour or unresponsive staring, may be present. The history and clinical observation of the patient's behaviour are usually sufficient for distinguishing true epilepsy from pseudoseizures. However, in difficult cases additional investigations, such as the measurement of post-ictal prolactin levels (which increase in most patients after true seizures) and/or EEG video telemetry, may be necessary.

Treatment of epilepsy

Drug treatment of epilepsy is usually very effective. The following are general principles of epilepsy management, but treatment should be individualised to suit the patient's needs:

1. Because anticonvulsant therapy is usually required for many years or even for life, a firm diagnosis of epilepsy should be made before the start of drug treatment.
2. It is generally accepted that in the case of idiopathic epilepsy the first seizure should not be treated because some patients never develop another epileptic seizure.

3. Normalisation of sleep and reduction of alcohol consumption (or preferably abstinence from alcohol) are important for seizure control.

4. The selection of the anticonvulsant drug should be based on the type of epilepsy, the drug's adverse effects profile, co-morbidities and the cost of the drugs. There are a large number of antiepileptic drugs. The efficacy of most of the new drugs (which are not mentioned here) has not been compared with the established first-generation anticonvulsants and their long-term effects are still not known.

5. Treatment should always be started with a single drug (monotherapy) because more than 80% of patients respond to treatment with one anticonvulsant agent. Treatment should also be started with a low dose and the dose is gradually increased until seizure control is achieved or adverse effects develop.

6. If the first choice drug fails to control the symptoms or causes significant adverse effects, a second-line drug could be used instead (see table 3.2). The dose of the first drug should be reduced gradually and slowly while the new drug is introduced also gradually.

7. When the epilepsy is not adequately controlled with the optimal dose of a single drug and the patient's compliance with treatment is confirmed, another anticonvulsant may be added (combination therapy). A third drug is required in very few cases.

8. The combination of carbamazepine with phenytoin, lamotrigine, clonazepam, valproate, primidone and phenobarbital should be avoided.

9. Phenytoin, phenobarbital and lamotrigine have a long half-life, and usually one daily dose taken at night is sufficient. (Compliance with treatment is often better with a single daily dose than with multiple dose regimes.)

10. In all cases it is important to be aware of the possible interactions between the anticonvulsants and other drugs.

11. Frequent change of medication should be avoided and anticonvulsant drugs should never be stopped suddenly. Sudden withdrawal of these drugs may increase the frequency of seizures significantly or result in status epilepticus.

12. Good control of epilepsy during pregnancy is important for the mother and the foetus, and treatment of epilepsy should continue throughout pregnancy. Most first-generation antiepileptic drugs, including phenytoin, carbamazepine, primidone and phenobarbital, may cause foetal congenital malformations and neurodevelopmental delay. Valproate has the highest teratogenicity and should be avoided, if possible, during pregnancy. However, the risk of the teratogenic effect is reduced with monotherapy at the lowest effective dose. Pregnant women on anticonvulsant medication should take folic acid supplements. This reduces the risk of spina bifida.

13. Anticonvulsants may reduce the effectiveness of the oral contraceptive pill and patients should be advised accordingly.

14. In patients with liver disease levetiracetam is preferred to other anticonvulsant drugs, and carbamazepine and valproate are safer than most anticonvulsants in those with chronic renal failure. In patients with heart disease phenytoin, carbamazepine and lamotrigine should be avoided, especially when cardiac conduction abnormalities are present.

15. In patients with symptomatic epilepsy, treatment of the underlying disease is necessary.

16. Drug treatment of epilepsy should only be stopped after careful consideration and in consultation with the patient because of the risk of relapse. The optimal time to discontinue anticonvulsant drugs in adults is not known at present. However, there is good evidence from randomised controlled trials that in children the risk of relapse is low after two years without seizures except in those who had a history of status epilepticus, an abnormal interictal EEG, focal seizures, or frequent seizures before the start of treatment.

17. Routine monitoring of the antiepileptic drug levels is not necessary for the optimal control of seizures in most patients. However, it is useful when poor compliance with treatment or drug toxicity is suspected and also as a guide for dose adjustments, especially in cases of combination therapy.

18. Surgical treatment is an option to be considered in cases of severe chronic epilepsy resistant to drug therapy (see below).

Table 3.2

Some of the first- and second-line drugs for epilepsy monotherapy and their daily adult dose:

Seizure classification	First choice drug	Second choice
Tonic-clonic seizures	Valproate (1-2 g) Carbamazepine (0.8-1.2 g) Lamotrigine (100-200 mg)	Phenytoin (200-500 mg) Primidone (0.75-1.5 g) Phenobarbital (60-180 mg) Oxcarbazepine (0.6-2.4 g)
Absence (petit mal)	Ethosuximide (1-1.5 g)	Clonazepam Lamotrigine
Petit mal + grand mal	Valproate	Clonazepam Lamotrigine
Simple partial or secondary generalised	Valproate Carbamazepine Lamotrigine Oxcarbazepine	Clobazam (20-60 mg) Levetiracetam (1-1.5 g) Gabapentin (0.9-3.6 g)
Complex partial	Oxcarbazepine	Carbamazepine

Treatment of generalised convulsive status epilepticus (GCSE)

GCSE is a life-threatening condition that causes severe hypoxia, acidosis and other severe metabolic derangements. It requires referral to a specialist intensive care unit without delay. Prompt treatment of GCSE is necessary to reduce mortality or the risk of brain damage in those who survive. Different guidelines for the treatment of GCSE have been published. All share the same principles and probably produce similar clinical outcomes. The management regime described here is widely used in North America and Europe.

The principles of GCSE management are treatment of the precipitating factors, suppression of the seizures and life support measures. All of these interventions, which are summarised below, should be started at the same time and continued for as long as necessary:

1. Continuous EEG monitoring and monitoring of vital signs.
2. Identification and treatment of the precipitating factor.
3. The correction of hypoxia, hypotension, hypoglycaemia and electrolyte imbalance. Tracheal intubation and assisted ventilation may be required.
4. Immediate administration of a benzodiazepine to abort the seizures. Any of the following may be used: lorazepam IV (0.1 mg/kg body weight, maximum dose 4 mg), midazolam IM (0.2 mg/kg, to a maximum of 10 mg), or diazepam IV or rectal (0.15 mg/kg to a maximum of 10 mg). The dose of the benzodiazepine may be repeated after 5 minutes.
5. The benzodiazepine treatment is followed by the administration of an IV infusion of an antiepileptic drug, e.g. valproate IV infusion (20-40 mg/kg at a rate of 3-6 mg/min) or phenytoin (20 mg/kg, 50-100 mg/min). If despite the above treatment the seizures continue for a further 15-20 minutes, midazolam infusion (0.2 mg/kg at a rate of 2 mg/min) or propofol infusion (20 mcg/kg) should be considered.
6. The IV infusion of the maintenance antiepileptic drug should continue for 24-48 hours after the cessation of the epileptogenic discharge (as confirmed by continuous EEG) before it is slowly and gradually withdrawn.

Surgical treatment of epilepsy

Patients with refractory epilepsy (usually defined as poor response to at least two antiepileptic drugs) and a well-defined epileptogenic focus on MRI scans that concords with the seizure clinical type and the interictal EEG are likely to benefit from the surgical resection of the epileptogenic focus. Surgery is particularly effective in the treatment of mesial temporal lobe epilepsy associated with hippocampal sclerosis that is resistant to drug therapy. It often results in complete cessation of the seizures or significant reduction in the anticonvulsant medication needed to control the symptoms. Other surgical procedures for epilepsy include neurostimulation with an implantable device, e.g. vagus nerve stimulation or deep brain stimulation.

Epilepsy and driving a motor vehicle

People with epilepsy often seek advice about driving a motor vehicle. Legislation in relation to driving should aim to protect the public without imposing too many restrictions on those who suffer from epilepsy. At present, the law in the UK allows epileptics to drive a motor vehicle for personal use provided they have seizures only during sleep for at least three years, or they did not have unprovoked seizures for at least one year and continue to take anticonvulsant medication. However, to drive a heavy goods vehicle or a public transport vehicle they must have been free from seizures without treatment for a minimum of 10 years.

Prognosis

Long-term remissions have been reported in 65 to 85% of patients with idiopathic epilepsy treated with anticonvulsant drugs. In some patients the remission is permanent. Early response to treatment and few relapses in the first year after diagnosis are good prognostic signs. On the other hand, high seizure frequency before the start of anticonvulsant medication and during the first year of treatment are indicators of poor prognosis. Those with neurological deficits and epileptic encephalopathies of childhood also have a poor prognosis. It is also possible that spontaneous remissions occur in epileptics who have never received anticonvulsant treatment.

Epileptics have a much higher mortality risk than the general population. It has been estimated that idiopathic epilepsy shortens life expectancy by two years. Life expectancy in patients with symptomatic epilepsy depends on the underlying pathology and may be reduced by as long as 10 years.

The highest rate of death in idiopathic epilepsy is in the first two years after the first seizure, and its main causes are epilepsy itself, injury due to accidental falls and suicide. Sudden unexplained death in epilepsy (SUDEP) occurs in some patients. However, neither the frequency, nor the pathogenesis of SUDEP is currently known. Poor seizure control, nocturnal seizures and chronic, severe tonic-clonic seizures appear to be important risk factors.

CHAPTER 4

CEREBROVASCULAR DISEASE

Cerebrovascular disease is a leading cause of disability and death worldwide. The main disorders in this group of neurological disease are stroke, multi-infarct (vascular) dementia, spontaneous subarachnoid haemorrhage, and acute and chronic subdural haematoma.

Stroke

Definition and epidemiology

Stroke, also called a cerebrovascular event (CVE), is a focal neurological deficit that occurs suddenly and lasts more than 24 hours, or results in death, and can only be explained by vascular occlusion or haemorrhage. This condition is referred to as a transient ischaemic attack (TIA) when the symptoms resolve in 24 hours or less.

Stroke is the most common neurological disease worldwide and is a leading cause of death and long-term disability. The total annual incidence of stroke (i.e. first-ever stroke and recurrent stroke) in the UK is between 100 and 290 per 100,000 of the population. There are variations between countries in the age-adjusted incidence of stroke, which can be explained by ethnic, environmental and cultural behavioural differences in lifestyle and by socio-economic factors.

The incidence of stroke increases with increasing age and the risk of having a stroke doubles every 10 years after the age of 55. Men tend to have more strokes than women of the same age. Stroke in childhood and in young adults is relatively rare except in those with haemoglobinopathies, such as sickle cell disease.

Stroke risk factors

A stroke risk factor is a condition that predisposes to stroke and also predicts the recurrence of stroke in a person who had a previous cerebrovascular event. The main risk factors for stroke and TIA are old age; Afro-Caribbean, Japanese, or Chinese ethnic origin; hypertension; atrial fibrillation; diabetes mellitus; hyperlipidaemia; cigarette smoking; and severe carotid artery stenosis. Frequently, more than one of these factors are present in the same patient.

Aetiology of stroke

Stroke may be caused by arterial occlusion resulting from thrombosis or embolism, or by rupture of the arterial wall. Vascular occlusion with a thrombus or a thromboembolism is, by far, the most common cause of stroke and accounts for more than 80% of all strokes. Spontaneous intracerebral haemorrhage, excluding subarachnoid haemorrhage, is the cause in approximately 10% of cases. Other causes of stroke include infections of the central nervous system, severe systemic hypotension (especially in the presence of stenosis of the cerebral arteries), bleeding into a brain tumour, and spontaneous dissection of the carotid or vertebral artery.

The clinical features of stroke

Stroke may be clinically silent or may result in significant focal neurological deficits, or even death. In addition, dysphagia, fatigue, sleep disturbances and depression are common after stroke. The clinical features largely depend on the size and site of the infarct or haemorrhage and the condition of the collateral cerebral circulation. There is a good correlation between the clinical features of stroke and the vascular territory involved. Several stroke syndromes can be identified.

Stroke involving the middle cerebral artery (MCA) is common. The lenticulostriate branch of the MCA supplies the internal capsule, the corona radiata and part of the basal ganglia. The superficial branches supply the sensory and motor cortex (except the leg area), and the auditory and language areas. Consequently, MCA stroke typically results in hemiplegia (the arm is affected more severely than the leg), hemisensory loss and hemianopia. In addition, apraxia and aphasia are present with dominant hemisphere lesions and left hemispatial neglect, and constructional apraxia with non-dominant hemisphere stroke. By contrast, stroke in the anterior cerebral artery territory is rare and causes crural monoplegia (weakness of one leg) or hemiparesis that predominantly affects the leg.

The posterior cerebral artery supplies the occipital cortex, the medial structures of the temporal lobe and the thalamus. A stroke in this vascular territory causes a visual field defect (usually upper quadrantanopia) and other visual symptoms, including visual hallucinations in the blind fields, and various visual perceptual difficulties. Stroke of the thalamus may cause reduced arousal and motivation, impairment of memory and learning, blunted emotional responses, mild transient dysphasia and personality change. Few patients develop the thalamic pain syndrome, which consists of severe, burning unpleasant tingling sensations in the paretic arm and leg.

The clinical signs of brain stem stroke vary depending on the site and size of the lesion. Large brain stem strokes are rare and usually fatal. They result from occlusion of the basilar artery. Non-fatal basilar artery strokes cause the 'locked-in syndrome'. The clinical presentation consists of paralysis of all skeletal muscles except the extra ocular and eyelid muscles. In addition, the patient develops anarthria and dysphagia.

Lacunar stroke
Small infarcts due to occlusion of end arteries are known as lacunar infarcts (lacunes are deep, small cavities in the brain tissue), which frequently occur in the internal capsule, corona radiata, thalamus and pons. They are usually associated with cigarette smoking, long-standing hypertension and diabetes mellitus. A single lacunar stroke is usually asymptomatic, but multiple lesions may cause vascular dementia or 'vascular' parkinsonism.

Intracerebral haemorrhage
Spontaneous intracerebral haemorrhage (ICH) accounts for approximately 10% of all strokes. Poorly controlled severe hypertension is the most common cause of ICH. Other causes include bleeding disorders, ruptured arteriovenous malformations and anticoagulant drugs.

The most common sites of ICH are the putamen, thalamus, cerebral hemispheres (lobar haemorrhage), the pons and the cerebellum. The onset of ICH is usually sudden and the clinical signs (and prognosis) depend on the size and site of the bleed. The bleeding often extends into the ventricles and reaches the cerebrospinal fluid. Large haemorrhages frequently cause brain swelling and result in displacement of brain tissue, brain stem compression, coma and death.

In contrast to other locations, the signs of haemorrhage in the cerebellum typically evolve over several hours. The patient usually presents with a severe headache, repeated vomiting, vertigo and ataxia. Brain stem signs develop over the following hours as the haematoma enlarges.

The treatment of ICH is mainly supportive. Surgical evacuation of the haematoma may save life in some cases. The prognosis of large ICH is poor. The mortality in the acute stage is approximately 30% and those who survive usually become severely disabled.

Differential diagnosis of stroke

Conditions that may be confused with stroke include Todd's paralysis following an epileptic seizure, hemiplegic migraine, acute and chronic subdural haematoma, brain tumours and hypoglycaemic episodes.

Diagnostic investigations

The diagnostic investigations of a patient presenting with a possible stroke should include brain imaging to confirm the diagnosis and type of stroke (i.e. haemorrhagic or ischaemic), and tests to screen for stroke risk factors. In addition, baseline measurements of the renal and hepatic function and blood clotting are usually necessary to help with the selection of the dose and type of medication for patients who require drug treatment.

A computerised tomographic (CT) head scan without contrast enhancement is the first choice radiological investigation of stroke. However, CT is much less sensitive than magnetic resonance imaging (MRI), especially for small brain stem and cerebellar stroke. As shown in figure 4.1, the typical CT appearance of an acute cerebral infarct is a low attenuation area corresponding to a vascular territory with or without a mass effect, such as shift of the brain's midline structures, due to cerebral oedema. In contrast to infarcts, intracerebral haemorrhage results in high attenuation lesions (see figure 4.2).

Figure 4.1
CT head scan. Low attenuation lesion due to a large cerebral infarct

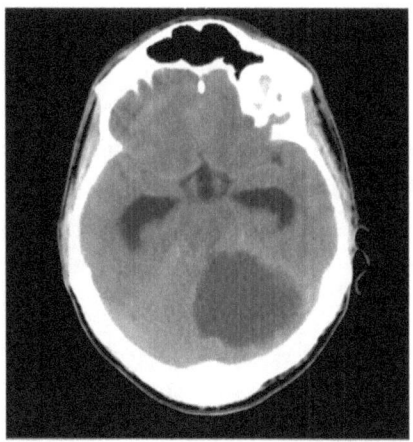

Figure 4.2
Ct head scan.
High attenuation lesion due to spontaneous intracerebral haemorrhage

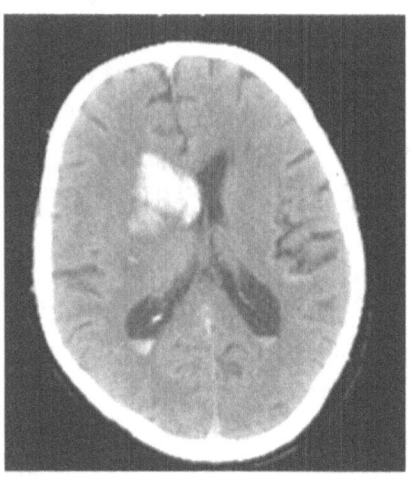

Spontaneous dissection of the carotid and vertebral arteries is a relatively common cause of stroke in young people. Non-invasive investigations, such as colour duplex ultrasonography, MRI scans and magnetic resonance angiography (MRA), are usually adequate for confirmation of the diagnosis, but cerebral angiography may be required in some cases.

All patients should also be screened for stroke risk factors. The diagnostic workup should routinely include measurements of blood glucose and serum cholesterol. In diabetics, the quality of glycaemic control should be established (by measuring the level of glycated haemoglobin – HbA1c). An ECG should be carried out to provide a record of the cardiac rhythm. Additional investigations are sometimes required when the less common causes of stroke are suspected.

Management of stroke
Medical care in the acute phase of stroke should aim to reduce mortality, to prevent or promptly reverse the early complications of stroke, and to create the optimal conditions for spontaneous and therapy-induced functional recovery.

Stroke leads to the development of an area of necrosis of brain tissue. Between the boundaries of this area and the intact brain tissue lies a zone of reduced cerebral blood flow known as the ischaemic penumbra. The residual perfusion in the ischaemic penumbra is largely dependent on the collateral circulation and the systemic blood pressure. The perfusion in the penumbral zone is just enough to support the basic cellular metabolic function for a few hours. However, complete recovery of the neurons in the ischaemic penumbra (and reduction of the neurological deficit) is often possible if the cerebral perfusion is restored quickly with therapeutic interventions, e.g. thrombolysis.

Thrombolysis is beneficial in some patients with mild or moderately severe ischaemic stroke. The thrombolytic agent currently used in stroke is alteplase or tissue plasminogen activator (tPA). Treatment with tPA is effective if the drug is given intravenously within approximately three hours of the stroke onset. The ischaemic aetiology of stroke must be confirmed with brain imaging and, in hypertensive patients, it is also essential to lower the systolic blood pressure to less than 185 and the diastolic to less than 110 mm Hg before the administration of tPA. The main complication of thrombolysis is bleeding. Thrombolysis is contraindicated in patients with a previous intracranial haemorrhage, myocardial infarction or severe traumatic brain injury in the three months preceding the stroke, major bleeding or surgery three weeks or less before the stroke, and early post-stroke epileptic seizures.

The clinical outcomes of stroke are improved when general supportive medical care is started promptly and the patient's condition is meticulously monitored. Steps should be taken to maintain nutrition and hydration, prevent hypoxia, control the arterial blood pressure, and to ensure the adequate treatment of hyperglycaemia and hyperpyrexia without delay (see table 4.1). Prevention of deep vein thrombosis and skin pressure sores is also an important aspect of acute stroke care.

Table 4.1
Summary of the main therapeutic interventions in acute stroke:

Symptom	Therapy intervention
Dysphagia	Dietary modification + IV fluid supplements if dysphagia is mild. In severe dysphagia start nasogastric tube feeding. If severe dysphagia persists 7 or more days, consider insertion of a gastrostomy tube.
Hypoxia	Oxygen saturation less than 95% – give oxygen by mask or nasal cannula. Consider assisted ventilation in cases of respiratory failure or severe cerebral oedema.
Blood pressure Systolic more than 220 or diastolic more than 120 mmHg	Empty bladder, treat constipation and pain, then observe. Treat hypertension if: a) patient is a candidate for thrombolysis, or b) there is evidence of hypertensive end organ damage.

Hypotension	Treat cause, e.g. volume depletion, arrhythmia, etc. Raise blood pressure to upper limit of normal with volume expanders and dobutamine.
Fever	Lower body temperature to normal.
Hyperglycaemia	Treat with insulin if blood glucose more than 16 mmol/L.

The secondary prevention of ischaemic stroke

A patient who has had a stroke or TIA is at risk of having another one in the future. The chance of recurrence is approximately 5-9% per year, and 1 in every 6 patients will have another stroke within 5 years of the index cerebrovascular event. Therefore, the overall management of stroke patients should include a strategy to reduce the risk of stroke recurrence by controlling the stroke risk factors and by the use of antithrombotic medication. Carotid endarterectomy is indicated in patients with severe internal carotid artery stenosis.

Aspirin (300 mg daily) is the antithrombotic agent of first choice. Treatment is normally started in the first 48 hours after stroke. Clopidogrel (75 mg once daily) is a suitable alternative in those who are allergic to aspirin or are unable to tolerate it. Patients on long-term treatment with aspirin who develop a further ischaemic stroke or TIA should be considered for combination therapy with aspirin 25 mg and dipyridamole MR 200 mg given twice daily.

Prognosis of stroke

The prognosis of stroke may be viewed in terms of the chances of surviving the acute cerebrovascular event, stroke recurrence and also the prognosis for functional recovery. All of these are influenced by the size and site of the stroke and the patient's previous health.

Mortality due to stroke is high, especially after spontaneous intracerebral haemorrhage. Between 20-30% of patients who are admitted to hospital with an acute ischaemic stroke die in the first 4 weeks. Early death after stroke is usually due to cardiac arrhythmias, massive pulmonary embolism, pneumonia, or brain stem compression due to extensive cerebral oedema.

The risk of stroke recurrence in the first 30 days is highest in patients with severe diabetes, congestive heart failure or a history of a previous stroke. Major stroke has an annual recurrence rate of 9%.

Approximately 80% of those who survive the acute cerebrovascular event regain some degree of independence with mobility and activities of daily living. Most of the functional improvement is usually achieved in approximately 3 months from the stroke onset. Predictors of poor functional recovery are old age, a severe initial motor deficit, poor sitting balance at 2-3 weeks, cognitive impairment, persistent apraxia, severe hemispatial neglect and Wernicke's aphasia.

Transient ischaemic attacks (TIAs)

TIAs result from embolism. In most cases, the embolus consists of platelets and fibrin material from an atherosclerotic plaque in the proximal segment of the internal carotid or vertebral arteries. Other sources of emboli include a mural cardiac thrombus, vegetations from cardiac valves and fragments of cardiac tumours, such as left atrial myxomas.

The clinical features of a TIA are similar to those of stroke but they resolve within 24 hours. Patients with a TIA are likely to develop a stroke in the future. Therefore, they should be routinely screened for stroke risk factors and any identified modifiable risk factors, e.g. significant carotid artery stenosis, should be treated. Long-term antithrombotic medication is also indicated.

Vascular dementia

Cerebrovascular disease is the third most common cause of dementia after Alzheimer's disease and Lewy body dementia. Vascular dementia (VD) mainly affects older people and its incidence progressively increases after the age of 75 years. Old age, hypertension, cigarette smoking and diabetes are the main risk factors for VD.

VD develops in patients with multiple lacunar infarcts in the cerebral white matter and basal ganglia. A lacunar infarct is the result of degenerative changes in the arterial wall of a single perforating artery and/or the formation of atherosclerotic plaques and in situ thrombosis.

Clinical features

The main clinical features of dementia, irrespective of its underlying aetiology, are gradual cognitive decline and changes in behaviour and personality. However, in contrast to Alzheimer's disease, the onset of VD is usually acute and its course is stepwise. Typically, the patient presents with mental confusion, impaired memory and concentration, and focal neurological signs followed by partial recovery. After a period of stable cognitive function, new neurological symptoms and signs develop and the cognitive deficits increase. This cycle is usually repeated several times during the course of the disease. The diagnosis of VD is confirmed by CT or MRI evidence of multiple lacunar infarcts in the basal ganglia and cortical white matter changes.

Treatment

Treatment of VD consists of the management of the stroke risk factors and the use of an antithrombotic agent. Cognitive rehabilitation is usually effective in the early stages of the disease.

Acetylcholine inhibitors, e.g. donepezil and rivastigmine, are effective in the treatment of mild to moderately severe Alzheimer's disease and dementia in Parkinson's disease. However, although postmortem studies have shown that VD frequently coexists with Alzheimer's disease, there is no sufficient evidence at present for the effectiveness of acetylcholine inhibitors in VD.

Subdural haematoma

A subdural haematoma (SDH) is a collection of blood between the dura mater and brain tissue. The bleeding results from a tear of one of the veins on the surface of the brain. These veins are known as the bridging veins and they are very susceptible to injury, especially when severe brain atrophy is present. SDH can be either acute or chronic.

Acute SDH results from severe head trauma and develops quickly resulting in compression of brain tissue, rise in the intracranial pressure and loss of consciousness. Typically, there a time lapse between the head injury and the loss of consciousness – 'the lucid interval'. However, some patients are comatose from the outset. As a rule, cerebral contusions and other injuries are also present.

In contrast to acute SDH, chronic SDHs are common in alcoholics and elderly frail subjects. They usually result from recurrent minor head injuries and they develop gradually over weeks or even months. The clinical symptoms and signs depend on the size of the haematoma. Patients often present with mental confusion, drowsiness, headaches and dizziness. Focal neurological signs may be present.

The diagnosis of SDH is confirmed with a CT head scan. Treatment of small SDH is conservative, but large haematomas require craniotomy and evacuation of the blood clot. The prognosis of chronic SDH is usually much better than that of acute SDH.

Subarachnoid haemorrhage

Non-traumatic subarachnoid haemorrhage (SAH) is usually due to spontaneous rupture of a saccular (berry) aneurysm and leakage of blood into the subarachnoid space. (Berry aneurysms are thought to result from developmental or acquired weakness of the vascular wall.) The main risk factors for SAH are hypertension, cigarette smoking, excessive alcohol consumption and a family history of SAH. The peak incidence is between the ages of 30 and 50 years.

Clinical presentation

The onset of SAH is sudden with severe headache, vomiting, photophobia and neck stiffness. Loss or impairment of consciousness, epileptic seizures and severe mental confusion are common. Clinical examination confirms the presence of signs of meningeal irritation, e.g. Kernig's sign and Brudzinski's sign (see page 78). Focal neurological signs, e.g. third nerve palsy or hemiparesis, are often present. The diagnosis of SAH is confirmed with CT head scan or with the detection of red blood cells and xanthochromia in the CSF (if the CT scan is negative). Identification of the ruptured aneurysm is made with cerebral angiography, CT angiography or magnetic resonance angiography.

Management

Medical treatment consists of general supportive care and the administration of nimodipine. (Nimodipine reduces the vasospasm that occurs in SAH and improves the clinical outcome.) Surgical treatment of hydrocephalus (which is a common complication of SAH) is sometimes necessary.

Recurrence of SAH is common. There is a 20% chance of another bleed in the first 3 weeks and 50% chance at 6 months. Therefore, embolisation or surgical clipping of the aneurysm is indicated in all patients, except in those with very poor prognosis.

CHAPTER 5

PRIMARY AND SECONDARY HEADACHES

Headache is a common complaint. It has been estimated that headache is the sole reason for referral in 20-25% of patients who attend a neurology clinic. The causes of headaches are numerous. Some of them are relatively benign, but others are associated with significant morbidity.

Headaches are classified into primary (idiopathic) and secondary (symptomatic) headaches. The first group includes migraine, cluster headaches and tension headaches. Secondary headaches are due to systemic disease.

Migraine

Migraine is one of the most common neurological disorders. It affects 15% of the population. The disease is more common in women and tends to run in families. Genetic factors are important in migraine. A single gene mutation is responsible for familial hemiplegic migraine, while other types of migraine are due to a combination of genetic predisposition and environmental factors. Migraine usually starts in early life and remits or becomes less frequent in old age.

The aetiopathogenesis of migraine is not fully understood. It is thought that the symptoms result from excessive activation of brain stem trigeminovascular pain pathways and cortical neurons. The excessive activation is followed by cortical depression. The observation that the frequency of migraine attacks increases during the menstrual period, and reduces during pregnancy and after the menopause suggests that oestrogen levels also have an important role.

Migraine is classified into migraine with aura (classical migraine), migraine without aura, familial hemiplegic migraine, and ophthalmoplegic migraine. The disease can be either episodic or chronic. Chronic migraine is defined as 15 or more attacks every month for 3 months or more.

Clinical features

Classical migraine is preceded by a number of symptoms that immediately precede the onset of the typical headache. This is the migraine aura. It usually consists of flashing lights (teichopsia), perception of zigzag lines or stars, blind spots and tingling skin sensations. Very rarely focal muscle weakness or dysphasia may occur. The aura usually lasts 5-15 minutes and is followed by the headache. A migraine aura is reported in approximately 20% of cases.

The typical migraine headache is severe or moderately severe, throbbing in nature and affects one side of the head. The migraine headache often starts on waking up in the morning, it reaches its maximum intensity in about an hour and usually lasts between four hours and three days. In severe cases it interferes with activities of daily living. It is made worse by physical activity and is usually accompanied by nausea, vomiting, photophobia and intolerance of noise. Transient focal neurological signs are sometimes present, e.g. oculomotor nerve palsies in ophthalmoplegic migraine.

The diagnosis of migraine is clinical. However, brain imaging is indicated when migraine occurs after the age of 50 years for the first time or is accompanied by epileptic seizures or unexplained focal neurological signs. Other indications are recent change in the pattern of the attacks, e.g. the occurrence of vomiting de novo and an aura lasting one hour or more.

Differential diagnosis

The unilateral frontotemporal localisation of the headache, its throbbing nature and the effect of physical activity on its severity distinguish migraine from other common types of primary headache, e.g. tension headache, cluster headaches and medication overuse headaches. Secondary headaches, e.g. headaches due to sinusitis, dental disease or systemic infection, are usually easy to diagnose because of the associated symptoms and signs of their underlying cause.

Treatment

It is important to identify and avoid the factors that trigger the migraine attacks. These include excessive consumption of alcohol or caffeine, poor sleep pattern, stress, long exposure to bright light and reduced physical activity. The assessment of the frequency and severity of the disease (by keeping a headache diary), and its impact on the patient's quality of life is necessary to inform the clinical decision of whether prophylactic treatment should be considered.

The first-line treatment of an acute migraine attack is a simple analgesic, such as paracetamol. However, the combination of paracetamol, aspirin and caffeine is more effective. Non-steroidal anti-inflammatory drugs (NSAIDs) are also a useful first-line treatment. When nausea or vomiting is also present the addition of an antiemetic, e.g. metoclopramide, is usually necessary.

The triptans, e.g. rizatriptan (10-20 mg/day), sumatriptan (200-300 mg/day) or zolmitriptan (7.5-10 mg/day), are usually effective when the first-line drugs fail to control the symptoms. The triptans are contraindicated in patients with uncontrolled hypertension, ischaemic heart disease and severe renal or hepatic failure, and during pregnancy. Ergot alkaloids (e.g. ergotamine 1-2 mg per day, maximum dose 4 mg) are also used, but they are less effective than the triptans. Opiates should be avoided in the management of migraine.

Prophylactic treatment is indicated in patients with chronic migraine (as defined earlier). Treatment is started with either topiramate (100 mg/daily), a beta blocker (e.g. propranolol 80-240 mg/day) or amitriptyline. If these drugs are ineffective, second-line drugs should be considered. These include valproate and calcium channel antagonists, such as flunarizine. In recent years, botulinum toxin injections into the faciocranial and cervical muscles have proved effective in the treatment of chronic migraine, although the mechanism of action is not known. Treatment with botulinum toxin is indicated if three or more of the above drugs have failed to adequately control the migraine attacks. Occipital nerve stimulation is also effective in some cases of refractory chronic migraine.

Cluster headaches

In contrast to migraine, cluster headaches are rare and most common in men and patients with multiple sclerosis. They are characterised by frequent, very severe unilateral headaches and autonomic disturbances. Cluster headaches are usually an episodic illness with remissions of a month or more between attacks. However, there is also a chronic form characterised by attacks that last more than one year without a remission of a month or longer. The disease onset is usually between the ages of 20-40 years. Occasionally cluster headaches are reported in patients with pituitary tumours and internal carotid artery dissection.

The cause of cluster headaches is not known, but genetic and environmental factors appear to be important. Heavy cigarette smoking and excessive consumption of alcohol are risk factors for cluster headaches. The current evidence suggests that the symptoms are due to hyperactivity of the trigeminal nerve pathways and the hypothalamus.

Clinical features

The headache often occurs at night usually 1-2 hours after the patient has fallen asleep. It is very severe, unilateral, and is orbital, periorbital or temporal. The headaches recur every night or every day for several weeks, and then stop for a variable length of time. The attack lasts from 15 minutes to 3 hours each time and may occur several times in one day. Excessive facial sweating, lacrimation, rhinorrhoea, nasal congestion and unilateral conjunctival injection are common associated features. Ptosis and miosis (partial Horner's syndrome) are frequently present and eyelid oedema may also occur. Frequently the patient is restless and agitated during the attack.

Treatment

Sumatriptan (6 mg by subcutaneous injection) usually relieves the symptoms of the acute attack in 15 minutes, especially if combined with the inhalation of oxygen by facial mask (100% concentration with a flow rate of 7 litres/minute). Intranasal sumatriptan is also effective. Verapamil (240-480 mg/day) is used for prophylaxis of cluster headaches. Lithium and topiramate are second-line drugs. Block of the greater occipital nerve and deep brain stimulation should be considered in chronic cluster headaches refractory to treatment.

Tension headaches

Tension headache is the most common primary headache. It occurs in all age groups and with similar frequency in both sexes. Its cause is not fully understood. However, it is thought that the disease results from increased activation of the pain receptors in the neck and craniofacial muscles, and the abnormal central processing of pain stimuli. Genetic susceptibility also appears to be important.

The headache is occipital or bilateral. The patient usually complains of a 'tight band', dull ache or pressure. The headache tends to occur during the day and lasts four hours or more. It is not accompanied by nausea, vomiting or photophobia. Typically, it is not made worse by physical activity.

Tension headaches should be differentiated from headaches due to neck arthritis, headaches that are associated with eye strain, diseases of the paranasal sinuses and dental disease. Treatment of the acute attack is with paracetamol and/or a non-steroidal anti-inflammatory drug. Amitriptyline may be used for prophylaxis.

Medication overuse headaches

Medication overuse headaches are defined as headaches associated with the frequent (more than 10 days per month) and inappropriate use of analgesic drugs. The treatment is often prescribed for an episodic headache, but the patient continues to take it for long periods and in large doses. As a result, the episodic headaches become chronic or more severe as a vicious cycle develops, i.e. continuous worsening of the headaches and progressive escalation of the analgesic medication dose. Medication overuse headaches are common in patients with psychiatric illness, especially mild and moderately severe depression and anxiety disorders.

Medication overuse headaches are usually similar to tension headaches. The diagnosis is based on the history of analgesics overuse and exclusion of the other types of primary and secondary headaches (table 5.1).

The treatment of medication overuse headaches consists of managing the precipitating and aggravating factors, treatment of the underlying disease and the gradual withdrawal of analgesic medication.

Table 5.1
Summary of the clinical features of the primary headaches:

Diagnosis	Highest incidence	Usual time of occurrence	Clinical features
Migraine	Females	Early morning	Aura Frontotemporal, unilateral Throbbing Nausea, photophobia
Cluster headaches	Males	At night, during sleep	Periorbital, unilateral Very severe Autonomic symptoms and signs
Tension and medication overuse headaches	No gender differences	During the day	Occipital or bilateral Like 'tight band' or dull No nausea or photophobia Worsened by exertion

Secondary headaches

Secondary headaches are very common. Most acute illnesses cause headaches that are resolved by successfully treating the underlying disorder. However, some secondary headaches are a sign of serious disease and require a further diagnostic workup and specific treatments. These are thunderclap headache, the headache of raised intracranial pressure, the headache of low CSF pressure, and temporal arteritis.

Thunderclap headaches
Thunderclap headache is a very severe and sudden headache that reaches its peak in one or two minutes. Although it is often described as pathognomonic of aneurysmal subarachnoid haemorrhage, it is frequently

caused by other disorders. These include vertebral or internal carotid artery dissection, hypertensive encephalopathy, venous sinus thrombosis, and intracranial hypotension due to low CSF pressure. An idiopathic form of thunderclap headache associated with reversible cerebral vasoconstriction is sometimes triggered by sexual intercourse (coital headache) and physical exertion.

Headaches of raised intracranial pressure
Raised intracranial pressure is most frequently caused by brain swelling, intracranial mass lesions (e.g. brain tumours, brain abscess, cerebral granulomas), venous sinus thrombosis and obstruction of the CSF pathways. Rarely, it is due to idiopathic benign intracranial hypertension. The main features of raised intracranial pressure are headache and visual symptoms.

The headache is usually persistent, non-pulsatile, diffuse or retro-orbital. Typically, it is worse in the early morning and improves as the day progresses. Activities that increase the intracranial pressure, such as coughing, sneezing and bending down, tend to aggravate the headache. Visual symptoms, including transient visual loss, scotomas and diplopia, are common. Vomiting occurs in severe cases. Some patients report dizziness or tinnitus. Focal neurological signs are often present on clinical examination (except in cases of idiopathic intracranial hypertension). Signs of papilloedema (raised pink optic disc with blurred margins, engorged retinal veins and retinal haemorrhages) are invariably seen on fundoscopy. Brain imaging usually reveals the underlying pathology.

On rare occasions the headache is due to idiopathic (benign) intracranial hypertension. This disorder predominantly affects young, obese women. Neurological examination is normal except for the presence of papilloedema. The CSF opening pressure is in excess of 200 mm H_2O, but the fluid is otherwise normal. Brain scans are also normal except for an empty sella turcica and an optic nerve sheath filled with CSF.

Treatment of raised intracranial pressure headaches depends on the underlying cause. For example, improvement in the symptoms of idiopathic intracranial hypertension may be achieved with reduction of body weight. If unsuccessful, treatment with acetazolamide (1-2 g/day) or topiramate is indicated. In severe cases, e.g. refractory headache or severe visual symptoms, insertion of a ventriculoperitoneal shunt or fenestration of the optic nerve sheath should be considered.

Headaches due to intracranial hypotension
CSF leaks following skull fractures or a lumbar puncture and low CSF volume due to over draining ventriculoperitoneal shunts are thought to result in headaches by causing traction on the meninges and the other pain-sensitive intracranial structures. In some cases, structural abnormalities of the meninges cause spontaneous CSF leaks.

Spontaneous low CSF pressure headache is more common in women and usually occurs between the ages of 50 and 60 years. The onset of the headache may be gradual, subacute or sudden (thunderclap). The headaches are typically affected by posture. They are triggered by standing up and improve or completely cease on lying down. They are usually accompanied by other symptoms, e.g. dizziness, blurring of vision, visual field loss, diplopia, limbs paraesthesia, nausea and neck pain. The opening CSF pressure is low (less than 60 mm H_2O). The CSF cell count, protein and glucose are normal.

The clinical diagnosis is confirmed by the typical appearance of gadolinium MRI head scan showing diffuse meningeal enhancement, subdural collection of fluid and downward displacement of brain structures.

Treatment of low pressure headaches depends on the cause of the CSF leak. Surgical repair is often required in cases of dural tears resulting from skull fractures. Post-lumbar puncture headache is self-limiting and responds to bed rest and hydration. Shunt revision is often indicated in cases of an over draining shunt. The first-line treatment of spontaneous CSF leak is epidural blood patching (the patient's blood is injected into the epidural space so that the blood clot plugs the leak). Surgical repair may be necessary if this procedure fails to stop the CSF leak.

Temporal arteritis

Temporal arteritis (also known as giant cell arteritis or cranial granulomatous arteritis) is a systemic autoimmune disorder characterised by the inflammation of medium and large arteries. The arteries that are most commonly affected by temporal arteritis are the branches of the external carotid artery and, less frequently, the aorta. The disease is more common in females and it rarely occurs before the age of 60 years. Patients with temporal arteritis also frequently have polymyalgia rheumatica, and vice versa.

Clinical features

The main symptoms of temporal arteritis are headaches, scalp tenderness, jaw claudication (pain in the jaw muscles caused by chewing), diplopia and sudden blindness. When polymyalgia rheumatica is present, there is also weakness and wasting of limb girdle muscles, weight loss, malaise and low-grade fever.

The headache is usually in the temporal region and can be either unilateral or bilateral. It is often persistent and dull, but is sometimes described by patients as burning. It can also be throbbing in quality. In some patients the temporal arteries are visibly thick and tortuous.

The erythrocyte sedimentation rate (ESR) and the C-reactive protein (CRP) are invariably raised. Duplex ultrasound and magnetic resonance angiography are useful insofar as they demonstrate thickening of the arterial wall, but their findings are not diagnostic. The definitive diagnosis is confirmed with temporal artery biopsy, which shows arterial wall thickening and infiltration with lymphocytes, macrophages and multinucleated giant cells.

Management

Temporal arteritis is a serious illness. Delay in treatment can cause permanent blindness due to ischaemic optic neuritis or central retinal artery occlusion. Therefore, treatment with high-dose steroids should be started immediately if the diagnosis is suspected.

The treatment of first choice is prednisolone (1 mg per kg body weight to a maximum of 60 mg/day) for at least 1 month. The headaches are usually relieved within 1 or 2 days of the start of treatment. The response to treatment is best monitored by its effect on the symptoms, and the ESR and CRP. Slow and gradual tapering of the dose (as guided by the ESR and CRP) to a maintenance dose (usually 5-10 mg of prednisolone/day) should be commenced after the first month of treatment. Early dose reduction may result in a relapse of the symptoms. Maintenance steroid treatment is recommended for at least two to three years. A bisphosphonate (e.g. disodium etidronate 200 mg/day) and a proton pump inhibitor (e.g. omeprazole 10 mg/day) should be prescribed together with the steroids to protect against osteoporosis and gastritis, respectively. Methotrexate is used when steroids fail to control the symptoms.

CHAPTER 6

INFECTIONS OF THE NERVOUS SYSTEM

Numerous micro-organisms can cause infection of the brain and spinal cord. These include bacteria, fungi (e.g. Cryptococcus), mycobacteria, parasites (e.g. cysticercosis) and viruses. Bacterial infections tend to cause acute illness, while fungal and mycobacterial infection usually results in subacute and chronic meningitis and encephalitis.

Acute bacterial meningitis

Acute bacterial meningitis is a serious infection of the leptomeninges (the arachnoid and pia mater), the ependyma and choroid plexus. It is most commonly caused by pneumococcus, meningococcus or haemophilus influenza species. In most cases, the bacteria reach the CNS by haematogenous spread from the upper respiratory tract, but the mechanism by which the bacteria breach the blood-brain barrier is not fully understood. Direct penetration, e.g. through bone defects due to skull fractures (especially basal skull fractures) or from an infected external ventricular drainage (EVD) shunt, also occurs.

Bacterial meningitis occurs either sporadically or in epidemics. Its highest incidence is in infants and young children.

Clinical features

The patient's initial presentation is usually with high fever, headaches, photophobia and vomiting. In severe cases stupor or coma are early features. Some patients also develop epileptic seizures early in the course of the disease. On clinical examination the patient is febrile and often agitated, irritable or drowsy. Neck stiffness and Kernig's sign and Brudzinski's neck sign of meningeal irritation are present.

The signs of meningeal irritation are due to inflammation of the spinal nerve roots. Kernig's sign is present when knee extension by the examiner beyond 135 degrees induces severe pain in a patient who is lying supine with his hips and knees flexed at 90 degrees. Brudzinski's neck sign is considered a more reliable sign of meningeal irritation than Kernig's sign. The test is also performed with the patient in the supine position. The examiner holds the patient's head with one hand and puts his other hand on the patient's chest to prevent the patient from rising. The examiner then raises the patient's head. This results in flexion of the patient's legs at the hips and knees when meningeal irritation is present.

Diagnosis
A lumbar puncture should be carried out immediately once meningitis is suspected. The pressure of the CSF at the start of the lumbar puncture is high and the fluid is turbid. On examination of the CSF there is a high white cell count (mainly neutrophils), high protein and reduced glucose. A Gram stain and CSF culture often confirm the diagnosis. The bacteria are also frequently found in blood culture.

The enzyme-linked immunosorbent assay (ELISA) for the detection of bacterial antigens is a useful diagnostic test when no organism is found on Gram stain and culture. Brain imaging is indicated when signs of raised intracranial pressure are present.

Treatment
Treatment of bacterial meningitis should be started as soon as possible even before the definitive confirmation of the diagnosis. It has been shown that delay of treatment beyond the first hour of the onset of symptoms increases mortality and the risk of the neurological complications. CSF and blood samples should be collected for culture and sensitivity testing before the start of the antibiotic therapy.

Treatment should be started with intravenous benzyl penicillin (2.4 g every 4 hours) or a broad spectrum cephalosporin, e.g. cefotaxime (2-4 g every 8 hours). In some cases, it is necessary to change the antibiotic according to the CSF culture and sensitivity results when these become available. Treatment should be continued for 10-14 days.

Life support measures and symptomatic treatment are required in addition to the antibacterial treatment. Corticosteroids, e.g. dexamethasone 0.6 mg/kg body weight daily for 4 days, are used to supress the inflammatory response. However, the current evidence suggests that corticosteroids do not have a significant effect on the mortality rate of severe bacterial meningitis, but they reduce the neurological complications, especially hearing loss.

Prognosis

The complications of bacterial meningitis in the acute stage include cerebral venous sinus thrombosis, cerebral oedema and raised intracranial pressure. Sensorineural deafness and epileptic seizures are usually late complications.

Bacterial meningitis has a high mortality rate. Approximately 10% of patients die despite receiving treatment with the appropriate antibiotics. The common causes of death are sepsis, brain stem compression due to cerebral oedema, and cardio-respiratory arrest. The prognosis of bacterial meningitis is influenced by the patient's age and the severity of the initial symptoms. Infants and older patients have a poor prognosis. Similarly, coma or reduced level of consciousness, early epileptic seizures, focal neurological signs, and very high protein or very low glucose in the CSF are poor prognostic signs.

Prophylaxis

Prophylaxis with antibacterial drugs (e.g. with rifampicin 600 mg twice daily for 2 days) reduces the risk of meningitis in close contacts of an index case. However, antibiotic prophylaxis of meningitis in patients with skull base fractures has no value, irrespective of the presence or absence of CSF leak.

Vaccination against some strains of meningococcus, pneumococcus and haemophilus influenza has been shown to significantly reduce the incidence of bacterial meningitis.

Tuberculous meningitis

The incidence and prevalence of tuberculous meningitis (TBM) depends of the frequency of the disease in the community and is also influenced by socio-economic factors and genetic susceptibility. The disease is more common in developing countries. In high-income countries it mainly affects immunocompromised individuals.

Tuberculosis is caused by the acid-fast bacillus Mycobacterium tuberculosis. The micro-organisms are thought to reach the CNS by haematogenous spread during the initial bacteraemia of the primary (usually pulmonary) infection. They may cause TBM at this stage or remain dormant. Activation of the latent infection may occur months or years later. The infection may cause any of the following: diffuse meningitis, cerebral vasculitis resulting in multiple infarcts, granulomas (a granuloma is a mass consisting of collagen, macrophages and other inflammatory cells), or solitary or multiple well-defined tuberculomas that are indistinguishable from other space-occupying lesions. Hydrocephalus and tuberculous encephalopathy (cerebral oedema, myelin loss and grey matter changes) also occur in the chronic stage.

The initial symptoms of TBM are usually non-specific and include general malaise, headaches and irritability. After 2-3 weeks these symptoms are usually followed by those of meningitis. Cranial nerve palsies, focal neurological signs and seizures are common. Hydrocephalus, encephalopathy or a large tuberculoma cause symptoms of raised intracranial pressure. Although the course of TBM is often subacute or chronic, occasionally the clinical presentation is acute and resembles that of bacterial meningitis.

The early diagnosis of TBM is difficult. The CSF protein and white cell count (lymphocytes) are raised and glucose is reduced. However, the CSF may be normal. Ziehl-Neelsen staining for acid-fast bacilli is negative in most cases and CSF culture may take up to six weeks. Various immunoassays and polymerase chain reaction (PCR) detection of the mycobacterial DNA have been used, but they generally lack sensitivity. Evidence of tuberculosis on chest X-rays has been reported in approximately 50% of cases.

In all cases fungal meningitis and neurosyphilis should be excluded. Brain imaging (usually a CT or MRI head scan) is indicated when focal neurological signs or signs of raised intracranial pressure are present.

Various protocols exist for the treatment of tuberculosis of the CNS. A frequently used protocol is a combination of the following four drugs: rifampicin, isoniazid, pyrazinamide and streptomycin (or ethambutol). This treatment is given for three months, and rifampicin and isoniazid are continued for a further six months after this period. In patients with tuberculous meningitis who are HIV negative, the addition of corticosteroids reduces the mortality rate and the long-term neurological complications. Dexamethasone 12-16 mg/day for 3 weeks and gradual discontinuation over the following 3 weeks has been shown to reduce the complications of TBM. Treatment also includes the management of complications and general supportive measures.

Unfortunately, the success rate of treatment of TBM is low, partly due to the frequent delay in diagnosis and also because resistance to anti-tuberculous drugs is common, especially in developing countries. Mortality of TBM is 25% in HIV (human immunodeficiency virus) negative patients and nearly 70% in those with HIV. Poor prognostic factors include severe disease and focal neurological signs on presentation, and normal CSF or low CSF cell count.

Non-bacterial meningitis

Aseptic meningitis

Aseptic meningitis is non-purulent (sterile) inflammation of the meninges. It may be caused by viruses (especially enteroviruses, such as Coxsackie B viruses, echoviruses, mumps and herpes simplex virus type 2), malignancy and drugs. Drugs that cause aseptic meningitis are some non-steroidal anti-inflammatory agents (ibuprofen, naproxen), antibacterial drugs (trimethoprim, cephalosporins), immune suppressant drugs (methotrexate) and anticonvulsants (lamotrigine, carbamazepine).

The clinical features of aseptic meningitis are similar to those of other forms of meningitis, but are usually less severe. Non-neurological signs may be present depending on the aetiology of the meningitis. For example, in aseptic meningitis due to mumps virus, parotitis and orchitis are usually present. Genital herpes is common when meningitis is caused by herpes simplex type 2 infection.

The CSF is clear. Mild abnormalities of CSF glucose, protein and CSF white cell count may be present. However, the CSF is sometimes normal. Bacterial and fungal antigens are not detected in the CSF, and CSF bacterial and fungal culture is negative.

It is often difficult to distinguish aseptic from bacterial meningitis, but the measurement of CSF lactate concentration is usually helpful. A CSF lactate level less than 2 mmol/L supports the diagnosis of aseptic meningitis. (In bacterial meningitis it is usually more than 6 mmol/L.)

Aseptic meningitis is usually benign and self-limiting. Its management consists of treatment of the symptoms and of the underlying cause.

Fungal meningitis
Fungal meningitis due to Cryptococcus is most common in Africa and frequently affects patients with HIV or AIDS. It is also common in other groups of immunocompromised patients, e.g. alcoholics, cancer patients and also in those on chemotherapy.

The course of cryptococcal meningitis is usually subacute. The CSF abnormalities are often unremarkable, but the diagnosis can be quickly and reliably confirmed by the detection of the cryptococcal antigen using the lateral flow immunochromatographic assay (LFIA). However, CSF culture remains the gold standard test.

The first choice treatment of cryptococcal meningitis is a combination of intravenous amphotericin and oral flucytosine. The prognosis of cryptococcal meningitis is poor. The mortality rate is approximately 50%.

Herpes simplex encephalitis

Encephalitis is diffuse inflammation of the brain's parenchyma. In cases where the meninges are also affected, the condition is called meningoencephalitis. Many viruses cause encephalitis, including herpes simplex virus types 1 and 2, varicella zoster, mumps, measles and enteroviruses.

Herpes simplex encephalitis (HSE) is by far the most important type of viral encephalitis because, if untreated, it results in very high mortality or severe disability in those who survive. It is also relatively common.

In the vast majority of cases, HSE is caused by herpes simplex virus type 1. The pathogenesis of HSE is not fully understood. A generally accepted hypothesis is that following the initial infection, the virus spreads to the nervous system and remains dormant in the sensory ganglia. After a period of time, the dormant virus is reactivated and causes encephalitis characterised by oedema and areas of focal necrosis predominantly in the medial aspects of the temporal lobes and the orbital surface of the frontal lobe, the insula and cingulate gyrus.

Clinical features and investigations

The initial clinical presentation of HSE is acute with high fever, altered level of consciousness (mental confusion, delirium, drowsiness or coma) and epileptic seizures. Focal neurological signs and signs of raised intracranial pressure are common in severe cases. The diagnostic workup of HSE should include analysis of the CSF, brain imaging and electroencephalography (EEG).

The routine examination of the CSF is helpful, but there are no specific changes that distinguish HSE from encephalitis caused by other viruses. The CSF protein is raised and the glucose is either normal or slightly reduced. There is also lymphocytic pleocytosis. Detection of the virus DNA in CSF with the polymerase chain reaction (PCR) is the best available method for the confirmation of HSE. It has high sensitivity and specificity, and the result can be available in 6-8 hours. Since the introduction of PCR, diagnostic brain biopsy has become obsolete.

Brain imaging is also an important part of the diagnostic workup of HSE encephalitis, and MRI head scans are the investigation of choice. High intensity signals on T2-weighted MRI brain scans consistent with focal brain swelling are typically present in the temporal lobes and the orbital surface of the frontal lobe. In addition, MRI evidence of infarcts and haemorrhages may also be present.

EEG is also useful. Diffuse slow waves and sharp waves in the temporal lobe leads are typical findings in HSE.

Differential diagnosis *
HSE should be differentiated from other types of viral encephalitis, and also from encephalopathy and disseminated acute encephalomyelitis (see Chapter 8 on demyelinating diseases). In tropical countries, cerebral malaria and the African sleeping sickness (trypanosomiasis) should also be considered.

There are no clinical features or abnormalities in the CSF cell count, protein or glucose levels that are specific to HSE. However, the differentiation between HSE and some types of viral encephalitis can be made with the PCR examination of the CSF. The PCR test is currently available for the diagnosis of HSE, varicella zoster and Epstein-Barr viral infections.

Encephalopathy is a non-inflammatory diffuse brain disorder. It results from severe cerebral anoxia, ischaemia and metabolic changes. Renal and liver failure, malignant hypertension and toxic substances are common causes. The patient presents with an altered level of consciousness, which increases progressively over several days until he lapses into a coma. Fever, headaches and focal neurological signs are usually absent. The CSF and brain imaging are normal, but the EEG shows diffuse slow waves. The sharp waves over temporal lobe areas that are typical of HSE are absent. Blood tests usually confirm gross metabolic abnormalities.

Trypanosomiasis is a parasitic illness endemic in Sub-Saharan Africa. It is transmitted by the bite of the tsetse fly. The parasite reaches the CNS by haematogenous spread. In the early phase trypanosomiasis causes fever, headaches, myalgia, malaise, hypersomnolence, lymphadenopathy and hepatosplenomegaly. If untreated it causes severe encephalitis. The diagnosis is confirmed with serological tests (the detection of trypanosoma antigens) and by isolation of the parasite from fluid aspirated from the lymph nodes. Rarely, the parasite is found in the CSF.

Treatment and prognosis
HSE is a lethal illness and is best managed in an intensive care unit. The response to antiviral medication is relatively good when treatment is started early. In addition to the specific antiviral treatment, the symptomatic management of hyperpyrexia, seizures, metabolic and electrolyte disturbances, e.g. the syndrome of inappropriate antidiuretic hormone secretion, etc., is also necessary.

Deterioration in the patient's condition can occur very quickly and treatment with the antiviral agent, acyclovir, should be started as soon as possible. The daily dose of acyclovir is 30 mg/kg body weight given in 3 divided doses by intravenous infusion over 1 hour. Treatment should be given for 14 days.

The prognosis of HSE is poor. Mortality is 70% without treatment, and 1 in 3 patients die even with acyclovir treatment. Complete recovery is rare in cases of HSE. More than 50% of the survivors will have long-term severe neurological complications, such as severe amnesia, motor deficits, aphasia and epilepsy.

Neurosyphilis

Syphilis is a sexually transmitted disease caused by the spirochete Treponema pallidum. (Non-sexual transmission is very rare.) The incidence and prevalence of syphilis is higher in sex workers and human immunodeficiency virus (HIV) positive individuals. CNS invasion occurs in 35% of patients and is more common in those with HIV infection, presumably because of their reduced immunity.

The clinical course of syphilis may be viewed in three distinct stages: primary, secondary and tertiary. Primary syphilis is characterised by the development of a painless ulcerating lesion (the primary chancre) on the external genitalia. When the disease is acquired through oral or anal sex the primary chancre develops on the lips, tongue or rectum. In addition to the primary chancre, regional lymphadenopathy is always present. The primary chancre heals spontaneously, but the secondary stage usually starts 2-3 months later.

The clinical features of secondary syphilis consist of fever, headache, general malaise, poor appetite, generalised lymphadenopathy and a generalised maculopapular skin rash, which is also present on the oral mucosal membranes. The clinical symptoms of untreated secondary syphilis also resolve in a few weeks, although recurrence may occur in the first two years after the primary infection. The CSF cell count and protein content are raised and the treponema is present in the CSF, but the patient does not have neurological symptoms or signs (latent neurosyphilis). The treponema invades the CNS usually in the first few weeks or months after the primary infection and remains dormant. The clinical manifestations of tertiary syphilis occur much later. For example, it has been estimated that in 25% of cases, tertiary syphilis develops after 8-10 years and the number of cases increases to 70% after 30-40 years of the initial infection.

Tertiary syphilis mainly affects the nervous system and the cardiovascular system (aortic aneurysms, aortic incompetence, etc.). The clinical manifestations of tertiary syphilis are meningovascular syphilis, general paresis, optic atrophy and tabes dorsalis. These are caused by various combinations of the following pathological changes: inflammation and thickening of the vascular wall and intra-arterial thrombosis, meningeal thickening, foci of cerebral infarcts, neuronal loss and white matter changes, brain atrophy, and obstructive hydrocephalus.

Meningovascular syphilis
The main clinical manifestations of meningovascular syphilis are meningitis, cervical pachymeningitis and meningomyelitis.

The onset of syphilitic meningitis is typically subacute and its course is chronic. Cranial nerve palsies and other focal neurological signs, and raised intracranial pressure are common in addition to the classical symptoms of meningitis. Recurrent stroke is an important feature of meningovascular syphilis. In contrast to tuberculous and pyogenic meningitis, constitutional symptoms are mild or absent and the patient is usually afebrile.

Cervical pachymeningitis is a combination of cervical radiculopathy and slowly progressive spastic tetraparesis. When the syphilitic pathological changes occur predominantly in the thoracic spinal cord, the patient presents with spastic paraparesis due to meningomyelitis.

General paresis
General paresis (or general paralysis of the insane) usually occurs 30-40 years after the initial infection and results from infection of the brain parenchyma. The patient presents with symptoms of progressive dementia and various focal neurological signs. The cognitive symptoms, at least initially, are not different from those of dementia due to other causes. However, some patients develop grandiose delusions and other psychiatric symptoms, such as paranoia and hallucinations. In the final stage of the disease, the patient becomes bedridden due to advanced paralysis. Death usually occurs 3-4 years after the onset of dementia.

Tabes dorsalis
In tabes dorsalis, the pathological changes are predominantly in the posterior columns of the spinal cord. The patient typically presents with sensory ataxia and positive Romberg's test. Brief, recurrent sharp pain that mainly affects the legs and may last several hours or even days occurs in almost all patients with tabes dorsalis. In addition, intermittent attacks of severe epigastric pain, colic and a feeling of constriction in the chest are also common and are generally known as visceral crises. The sensory loss leads to the development of trophic ulcers in the feet and a painless arthropathy (Charcot's joints), which most commonly affects the knees. Argyll Robertson pupils (symmetrical small pupils that do not react to light, but constrict on accommodation) are typical signs of all forms of neurosyphilis.

Laboratory diagnosis of neurosyphilis

The clinical diagnosis of neurosyphilis is primarily confirmed with the standard examination of the CSF and serological tests. Brain imaging is also useful in most cases.

The CSF contains an increased number of cells (mostly lymphocytes), increased protein and normal glucose. The CSF serological tests are also positive. A combination of a treponema-specific and a treponema-non-specific serological test should be used.

A positive fluorescent treponema antibody-absorption test in the CSF sample confirms the diagnosis of neurosyphilis, but it does not distinguish active from non-active disease. To assess the disease activity a treponema-non-specific, quantitative test is required. The Venereal Disease Research Laboratory (VDRL) test is the most widely used. Despite its low sensitivity as a diagnostic test, the VDRL test is useful for monitoring the disease activity and the response to treatment. High titres correlate with disease activity and the opposite is also true.

In patients with neurosyphilis, MRI brain scans often demonstrate evidence of vasculitis (focal areas of high signal intensity), meningeal enhancement, cerebral infarcts, and mild or moderately severe brain atrophy.

Treatment

Treatment of the early stages of syphilis with adequate doses of penicillin is curative. In late tertiary syphilis, treatment usually arrests the disease progression but does not reverse the existing neurological damage.

The drug of first choice is a single dose of benzathine penicillin G 2.4 million units given by intramuscular injection. Some clinicians recommend the administration of two more doses, one in each of the second and third weeks.

Procaine penicillin (penicillin G) may be used as an alternative to benzathine penicillin. The daily dose of procaine penicillin is 24 million units given by a single deep intramuscular injection and the duration of treatment is 10-14 days. Probenecid tablets (500 mg every 6 hours) are also given for the same duration in order to maintain a high concentration of penicillin in the CSF.

Oral doxycycline (100 mg twice daily for 14 days) is suitable for patients who are hypersensitive to penicillin. The response to treatment is monitored with VDRL CSF titres. A four-fold fall in titre at 6 months is considered evidence of a good response to treatment.

Human immunodeficiency viral infection of the nervous system

The human immunodeficiency virus (HIV) is a retrovirus that is acquired through unprotected sexual intercourse with an infected person, transfusion of contaminated blood or the use of contaminated hypodermic needles. Transplacental transmission also occurs. The spectrum of HIV infection ranges from initially mild disease to the severe, potentially fatal illness – the acquired immunodeficiency syndrome (AIDS). Patients with HIV infection are also susceptible to opportunistic infections and malignant tumours, e.g. Burkitt's lymphoma, Kaposi's sarcoma and primary CNS lymphoma. The disease is most common in Sub-Saharan Africa, in intravenous drug users and homosexual men.

The initial presentation of HIV infection is with transient flu-like symptoms after which the patient usually remains asymptomatic for a number of years. During this asymptomatic period, the virus continues to replicate and attack the immune system destroying CD4 T cells (T Helper lymphocytes). The clinical features of AIDS develop when the CD4 cell count falls to a critical number (usually less than 50 cells/mm^3). The patient presents with high fever, sweating, weight loss, gastrointestinal symptoms and generalised lymphadenopathy. Few patients also have a generalised maculopapular rash. The virus invades the CNS during the viraemia of the initial infection, but the neurological complications of HIV infections are usually delayed for a number of years.

The neurological complications of HIV/AIDS result either from the direct virus invasion of the CNS or from the effects of the virus on cell immunity.

119

The virus infects the microglia, macrophages and astrocytes, and causes inflammatory changes in the brain parenchyma and in the spinal cord, especially the posterior and lateral columns. It does not infect the nerve cells directly, and the neuronal damage is secondary to the effects of the disease.

The direct effect of the virus on the CNS causes acute and chronic meningitis, dementia, myelopathy and polyneuropathies. HIV infection also severely reduces cell immunity, which allows micro-organisms with normally low pathogenicity to cause serious illness, i.e. opportunistic infections. The low immune status also increases the patient's risk of acquiring other infections, e.g. tuberculosis or syphilis. Primary CNS lymphoma is also common in HIV-positive individuals. Metabolic encephalopathies due to systemic complications, such as anoxia resulting from severe respiratory infection, also occur.

Meningitis
Acute meningitis is common in the early stage of HIV infection and may precede the other manifestations of the disease by a long period of time. It is a mild, self-limiting disease indistinguishable from other forms of aseptic meningitis either clinically or in terms of CSF abnormalities. Chronic meningitis also occurs and is asymptomatic in 40% of patients.

HIV-associated dementia
Before the anti-retroviral treatment became available, dementia was reported in two thirds of patients with AIDS. It is now less common in treated patients. However, milder forms of cognitive impairment are frequently present in successfully treated patients, especially in older subjects. The onset of dementia is insidious and its course is relentlessly progressive.

Clinically, HIV-associated dementia is similar to other types of subcortical dementia. It is characterised by the triad of diffuse cognitive impairment, focal motor system signs (ataxia, tremor, myoclonus, spastic paraparesis) and behavioural disturbances, such as loss of spontaneity and apathy. Brain imaging demonstrates diffuse white matter changes and cerebral atrophy.

Myelopathy

Typically the onset of myelopathy is gradual. The clinical presentation is that of slowly progressive asymmetrical spastic paraparesis, sensory ataxia, muscle cramps, sensory loss and paraesthesia in the lower limbs, and loss of bowel and bladder control.

Peripheral neuropathy

HIV peripheral nervous system disease causes demyelinating polyneuropathy (similar to Guillain-Barré syndrome), sensorimotor neuropathy and mononeuritis multiplex. Sensorimotor neuropathy is the most common of these disorders. It affects as many as 65% of patients in the later stages of AIDS.

Opportunistic CNS infections

The most common opportunistic infections in HIV/AIDS are toxoplasmosis, Cryptococcus and cytomegalovirus virus infection. Varicella zoster, candida, and listeria infections are less common. Opportunistic infections cause focal neurological deficits, encephalopathy and systemic symptoms, such as fever and headaches.

Toxoplasmosis

Toxoplasma gondii is a protozoan that infects warm-bloodied animals. The most important host of the toxoplasma is the domestic cat. The parasite multiplies in the gut of the cat and is excreted in the faeces. Infection is mainly due to ingestion of contaminated food or water. Like other opportunistic infections, toxoplasmosis does not cause serious disease except in immunocompromised patients. Brain imaging and serological tests are the main diagnostic investigations. The CT scan typically shows multiple lesions with or without ring enhancement in the cerebral cortex and basal ganglia. (Similar scan abnormalities are seen in some cases of primary CNS lymphoma.) The serological tests for toxoplasmosis (toxoplasma IgG antibodies) are positive in most cases. Treatment with a combination of pyrimethamine (200 mg loading dose, followed by 50 mg once daily) and sulphadiazine (1 g four times a day) usually results in clinical improvement within 24-48 hours. Folic acid (10 mg daily) should also be prescribed to reduce the toxicity of pyrimethamine.

Cryptococcosis

The fungal infection, cryptococcosis, (also known as cryptococcal disease) is acquired by the inhalation of the spores. Cryptococcal infection is usually asymptomatic in an immunocompetent individual, but it can also cause mild, self-limited respiratory infection and then becomes latent. The infection is reactivated when cell immunity is severely depressed. The diagnosis is confirmed by the identification of the cryptococcal antigen in the CSF with the latex agglutination test. The combined treatment with amphotericin B (0.7 mg/kg once daily) and flucytosine (25 mg/kg six hourly) for two weeks is usually effective.

Cytomegalovirus infection

Asymptomatic cytomegalovirus infection is very common worldwide. Reactivation of the latent infection may cause encephalitis, myelitis, radiculopathy, peripheral neuropathy and blindness due to chorioretinitis. A definitive diagnosis is made when the virus particles are detected in the CSF with the PCR test. Treatment is with intravenous ganciclovir (5 mg/kg twice daily).

Primary CNS lymphoma

Primary CNS lymphoma is a rare neurological malignancy (it accounts for only 2% of all brain tumours) except in the context of immunodeficiency. The tumour can cause focal signs in any part of the CNS, and the clinical presentation depends on the site of the lesion. A brain biopsy is required for a definitive diagnosis. The prognosis is generally poor, but combination chemotherapy, e.g. high dose of methotrexate and cytarabine, is effective in some patients.

Laboratory diagnosis of HIV infection

Various laboratory tests are used in the diagnosis and management of HIV infection. The standard method for the diagnosis of HIV infection is to use two serological tests together. Screening for HIV antibodies is first made with the enzyme-linked immunosorbent assay (ELISA). The result is confirmed with the Western Blot test.

The response to treatment is assessed by measuring the plasma HIV RNA levels, and CD4 T cell count is routinely used to monitor the patient's immune status and the risk of acquiring opportunistic infection.

CSF examination is also indicated for the diagnosis of opportunistic and other CNS infections, e.g. tuberculosis, syphilis and malaria, and in HIV meningitis.

Treatment

Early treatment of HIV infection with a combination of antiretroviral drugs is effective in most cases. In addition, treatment of the opportunistic infections and the management of symptoms are also necessary.

Many antiretroviral drugs are currently available. Combination antiretroviral therapy increases the patient's immunity, suppresses the viral replication and reduces the spread of the virus to the CNS. It is recommended that a combination of three drugs is used in the treatment of patients with CNS complications: the drug regime should include two of the nucleoside reverse transcriptase inhibitor drugs that have good CNS penetration (e.g. zidovudine and abacavir) and one of the protease inhibitors (e.g. ritonavir).

Prognosis

Successful treatment of HIV infection with antiretroviral drugs reduces mortality and prolongs the patient's survival. Nowadays, most treated patients have a normal or near-normal life expectancy. Treatment also reduces the incidence of opportunistic infections and improves the patient's health-related quality of life. However, it has limited impact on the neurological complications. This is probably due to the poor CNS penetration of most of these drugs, which allows the slow replication of the virus and persistence of the infection. The poor response of the neurological complications to treatment may also be due to the toxicity of the antiviral medication and/or other co-morbid conditions, such as coincidental cerebrovascular disease or Alzheimer's disease.

Without antiretroviral drug treatment the prognosis is poor. The average survival is 9-11 years from the date of the primary infection and is less than 2 years after the onset of AIDS.

Acute poliomyelitis

Acute poliomyelitis (polio) is an infection of the nervous system that is caused by the polio virus. There are three strains of the virus: one, two and three. In most cases the paralytic variant of polio is caused by type one virus. Thanks to successful worldwide vaccination programmes in the last few decades, endemic polio has now been eradicated. However, sporadic cases still occur.

The infection is acquired through the consumption of contaminated food or drink. The virus replicates in the gastrointestinal tract for 2-3 weeks and then enters the systemic circulation. In more than 90% of cases the viraemia is either asymptomatic or causes mild flu-like symptoms. However, in some patients it results in mild aseptic meningitis or paralytic polio.

In paralytic polio, the virus most frequently infects the motor neurons of the spinal cord, but it can also affect the brain stem. This causes an inflammatory reaction and necrosis of the anterior horn cells of the spinal cord and, in the case of brain stem infection, the bulbar neurons.

Clinical features of paralytic polio

The onset is acute with high fever, myalgia, headaches, diarrhoea and vomiting. Flaccid muscle weakness develops quickly and reaches its peak severity in 2-3 days. The paralysis is asymmetrical and is usually confined to the lower limbs.

The bulbar form of polio is usually severe. Dysphagia, dysphonia and respiratory muscle weakness develop after an initial prodromal phase of constitutional symptoms. Hypotension and other symptoms of autonomic dysfunction (e.g. gastroparesis) may also be present. However, limb weakness is rare.

Differential diagnosis

Polio should be differentiated from other conditions that cause acute flaccid paralysis, e.g. Guillain-Barré syndrome, polymyositis, botulism and West Nile viral infection. The clinical diagnosis of polio is confirmed by isolation of the virus. Serological tests have little value in diagnosis because the interpretation of these tests is difficult. They only provide information about the patient's immune status and do not distinguish newly acquired polio from a pre-existing immune response due to previous vaccination. Routine CSF analysis is also of limited diagnostic value. It shows a rise in protein and cell count (lymphocytes). The glucose is usually normal.

The diagnosis of polio is confirmed by the isolation of the virus from the culture of the patient's stools. The culture of 2 samples taken 24 hours apart in the first 4 weeks of infection are likely to confirm the diagnosis in nearly all cases. PCR of the CSF is another useful diagnostic test, when available.

Treatment and prognosis

There is no specific antiviral drug for the treatment of polio. The management is symptomatic with bed rest, pain relief, etc. Artificial ventilation may be required in cases of bulbar polio. Rehabilitation is the mainstay of management in the post-acute stage.

Severe polio, especially the bulbar form, is a potentially lethal illness. The mortality rate depends on many factors and varies from 5% in some countries to more than 30% in others. Complete recovery from severe polio is rare. In most cases residual muscle weakness causes long-term locomotor disability. Other late complications include skeletal deformities (scoliosis, kyphosis), and knee and hip joint instability. The post-polio syndrome is also common.

Post-polio syndrome (PPS)

PPS is a late complication of polio. It usually occurs 15 years or more after the initial infection. The cause of PPS is not known, although currently available evidence suggests that persistence of the polio virus and a low-grade infection may be responsible. The syndrome is characterised by the development of new focal muscle weakness and wasting after many years of stable neurological function. Generalised fatigue and myalgia are common. The diagnosis is made by excluding other causes of focal muscle atrophy. There is no effective drug treatment for PPS at present. Some functional improvement is often possible with intensive rehabilitation.

Protection against polio
The trivalent oral vaccine (which is made of live attenuated viruses) provides excellent protection against polio infection. However, there is a risk that it might lead to the emergence of new vaccine-derived polio viruses. The World Health Organisation has, therefore, recently embarked on a programme of gradually replacing the trivalent oral vaccine with an inactivated polio virus vaccine. The programme is scheduled to complete by 2019. Currently, clinical trials are being conducted to define the optimal dose and frequency of administration of the new inactivated vaccine and the child's age at which vaccination is most effective.

Herpes zoster
Herpes zoster (shingles) is a relatively common neurological disorder. Its estimated annual incidence is 3-4 per 1,000 of the general population. The incidence is significantly higher in older people and immunocompromised subjects (irrespective of their age).

Herpes zoster is caused by the varicella-zoster virus and, typically, develops many years after the patient has recovered from chickenpox. It is thought that at the time of infection with chickenpox, the virus migrates from the skin to the sensory ganglia via the axons of peripheral nerves and remains dormant in the ganglia, usually for many years. Activation of the virus occurs when the subject's cell immunity is reduced. The activated virus travels along the sensory nerve to the skin and causes the characteristic rash over one or more skin dermatomes.

Clinical presentation
Patients with herpes zoster present with a characteristic skin rash. The rash is usually preceded by local itching, tenderness and hyperaesthesia. Mild systemic symptoms, consisting of fever and malaise, are also present.

Initially the skin rash consists of erythematous papules. Within a day or two the papules evolve into vesicles and then pustules. By the end of the second week the pustules dry leaving a crust and, later, a scar.

The rash distribution corresponds to the dermatomes of one or more of the sensory nerves. Most frequently the rash occurs in the thoracic region. It is frequently unilateral, but may involve both sides of the body in immunocompromised patients.

Infection spreading from the trigeminal ganglion along the ophthalmic division of the trigeminal nerve (ophthalmic herpes zoster) occurs in approximately 20% of patients. The distribution of the skin rash is in the forehead. Ophthalmic herpes zoster often causes serious eye complications, including keratitis, conjunctivitis, iritis, scleritis and retinal necrosis.

Herpes zoster may also affect other cranial nerves. Ophthalmoplegia due to oculomotor nerves involvement and facial palsy accompanied by a vesicular rash in the external auditory canal (Ramsay Hunt syndrome) occur in some patients. Chronic radiculopathy without a skin rash has also been reported.

Diagnosis
It is not difficult to make a clinical diagnosis when the characteristic skin rash is present. However, in atypical cases confirmation of the diagnosis requires laboratory investigations. PCR is the most sensitive test. Alternatively, immunohistochemical analysis of skin scraping may be used.

Treatment and prevention
A systemic antiviral drug should be administered within 72 hours of the skin rash. Any of the following drugs may be used: acyclovir (800 mg five times/day), famciclovir (500 mg three times/day), or valacyclovir (1 g three times/day). The duration of treatment is 7 days (or 10 days in immunocompromised patients).

Vaccination should be considered in older people (over 60 years of age). The vaccine (live, attenuated virus) is effective in people who had no history of varicella-zoster infection. It also boosts the immunity in those with previous exposure to the virus.

Complications of herpes zoster

The most common complications of herpes zoster are post-herpetic neuralgia and segmental muscle weakness due to motor neuropathy. Other less common complications due to the reactivation of the varicella-zoster virus include meningoencephalitis, myelitis, stroke due to vasculopathy, and retinal necrosis.

Post-herpetic neuralgia is characterised by severe pain in a dermatomal distribution which is present for 90 days or more after the appearance of the skin rash. It affects 40% of patients. A severe skin rash, old age and depressed immunity are the main factors that predispose to post-herpetic neuralgia. The pain is usually a combination of constant severe, burning pain, and paroxysmal electric shock-like sensation. In addition, pain that is caused by a light touch of the affected skin is also common. The pain responds poorly to most analgesic drugs and is frequently associated with depression. Treatment with a local anaesthetic cream (e.g. lidocaine) or with capsaicin cream is usually sufficient in mild cases. In severe post-herpetic neuralgia, systemic medication is always required. Gabapentin, pregabalin and the tricyclic antidepressants result in partial or complete symptomatic relief in most cases.

Segmental muscle wasting and weakness usually occurs 2-3 weeks after the disease onset and corresponds to the dermatomal distribution of the skin rash, except in approximately 10% of cases. The muscle weakness is usually unilateral and frequently affects the cervical and lumbosacral region. Weakness of the diaphragm and abdominal muscles may also occur. The prognosis is usually good. As a rule, complete recovery occurs in 6-12 months in most cases.

Cerebral malaria

Malaria is a parasitic infection endemic in Sub-Sharan Africa and some parts of Asia. The parasite, plasmodium, is transmitted through the bite of infected female anopheles mosquitos. Four plasmodium species (vivax, malaria, ovale and falciparum) cause malaria in humans. However, only plasmodium falciparum causes cerebral malaria.

The pathogenesis of cerebral malaria is complex. During feeding, the mosquito ingests the sexual forms of the parasite from the blood of an infected subject. When the parasite is transmitted to a non-immune person, the plasmodium develops in the subject's liver for 2-3 weeks. It is then released into the circulation and invades the red blood cells. This causes the clinical signs which, in the case of falciparum malaria, normally last 48 hours. Severe parasitaemia, non-immune status, pregnancy and delay in treatment may lead to the development of cerebral malaria.

Postmortem studies in cases of fatal cerebral malaria have shown that the brain capillaries and venules are clogged up with the parasitised red blood cells and thrombi. This microvascular obstruction and changes in the vascular endothelium are thought to cause disruption of the cerebral microcirculation, ischaemic, hypoxic and metabolic changes, and coma.

Clinical features
Cerebral malaria is rare among adults in endemic areas because immunity is usually acquired through repeated mild infections by the age of 5 years. Sickle cell disease (which is common in Sub-Saharan Africa) also confers a protective effect against malaria. Therefore, most patients who develop cerebral malaria are very young children, non-immune travellers to endemic areas and immunocompromised subjects.

The patient usually complains of fever, sweating, rigors, vomiting and headaches for a few days. These symptoms are followed by jaundice, anaemia and convulsions, and mental confusion. Delay in treatment usually results in coma. Decerebrate or decorticate postures are common. Retinal haemorrhages and bruxism may be present.

The diagnosis is confirmed by the detection of the parasite in thin and thick blood films, and the exclusion of other causes of encephalopathy. In endemic areas, cerebral malaria should be excluded only after 3 negative blood films taken 8-12 hours apart.

Laboratory tests almost always show abnormal liver function, haemolytic anaemia, hypoglycaemia and impaired renal function. The ESR is raised. The CSF is clear. There is mild lymphocytic pleocytosis, normal protein and normal glucose. The CT head scan is normal, except when cerebral oedema is present and the EEG changes consist of non-specific generalised slow waves.

Treatment

Treatment consists of the prompt administration of specific anti-malarial drugs and the management of the acute complications of cerebral malaria. Adjunct corticosteroid treatment has no effect on the mortality rate and is associated with an increased risk of gastrointestinal haemorrhage and seizures.

Quinine has been used for the treatment of severe malaria, including cerebral malaria, for many decades. However, the artemisinin derivatives (artemether, arteether, artesunate and dihydroartemisinin) have proved to be as effective as quinine and have less adverse effects. Furthermore, in some areas the malaria parasite has developed resistance to quinine. Nowadays, artesunate is the drug of first choice for the treatment of cerebral malaria. It is given by intravenous injection in a dose of 2.4 mg/kg body weight twice daily on the first day, followed by 2.4 mg/kg once daily for another 6 days. Quinine should be used if the artemisinin drugs are not available.

Quinine loading dose (20 mg salt/kg body weight over 4 hours) should be given intravenously as soon as possible. Eight hours after the loading dose, treatment is continued with the intravenous infusion of 30 mg salt/kg per day. Quinine treatment requires careful monitoring as the drug may cause hypoglycaemia and hypotension.

The clinical outcome also depends on the timely and appropriate management of acute complications of cerebral malaria, including cerebral oedema, hypoglycaemia (especially when quinine is used because it causes insulin release from pancreatic cells), shock, hyponatraemia, acidosis, pulmonary oedema and acute renal failure.

Prognosis

Recovery from coma usually occurs in 48 hours with successful treatment, and long-term neurological complications are relatively rare. However, the mortality rate of cerebral malaria is high. Approximately 20% of treated patients die, and the risk is highest in children, pregnant women and those with no previous exposure to malaria.

Malaria prophylaxis

A non-immune person intending to travel to endemic areas should be advised to avoid mosquito bites and to take anti-malarial drugs for prophylaxis. The choice of drug depends on the area of the intended travel because the parasite's resistance to anti-malarial drugs varies from one country to another. The prophylactic treatment should be started two weeks before travel and continued for four weeks after return from the endemic area.

CHAPTER 7

EXTRAPYRAMIDAL DISEASE

The extrapyramidal system (basal ganglia) consists of the caudate nucleus, putamen, substantia nigra and the subthalamic nucleus. Diseases of the basal ganglia result in abnormalities of movements, posture and righting reflexes without causing significant focal muscle weakness. The most common extrapyramidal disorders are tremor, Parkinson's disease, dystonia and blepharospasm. Other manifestations of basal ganglia disease are chorea, athetosis, myoclonus and tics. However, these are usually features of other diseases rather than separate clinical entities.

Tremor

Tremor is defined as involuntary rhythmic regular movements of any part of the body. It is more common in the limbs and head and, when severe, it causes difficulties with handwriting and various activities of daily living. Voice tremor may interfere with vocalisation. Tremor is classified into rest, action, intention, and dystonic tremor. While this classification is useful in the diagnosis and treatment, pure forms of tremor are rare in practice.

Rest tremor is a characteristic sign of Parkinson's disease. It is usually unilateral and, in most cases, affects the hand. Typically, the thumb beats against the index finger (hence it is frequently described as bead rolling or pill-rolling tremor). The severity of the tremor increases with anxiety and diminishes during voluntary movements of the affected limb. It disappears during sleep. Other features of parkinsonism, e.g. bradykinesia and muscle rigidity, are invariably present.

Action tremor is fine tremor that is present throughout the range of voluntary movement. It is often caused by overactivity of the sympathetic nervous system, as occurs in thyrotoxicosis and alcoholism. Numerous drugs also cause action tremor. Examples are sympathomimetic and antimuscarinic bronchodilators (salbutamol, terbutaline, aminophylline), tricyclic antidepressants (amitriptyline, clomipramine), selective serotonin reuptake inhibitors (citalopram, fluoxetine, paroxetine) and anticonvulsants drugs (lamotrigine, levetiracetam).

Intention tremor is characterised by an increase in amplitude as the limb approaches the target, e.g. during the performance of the finger–nose test. It is due to cerebellar disease. In addition to intention tremor, the patient usually has ataxia, nystagmus, dysarthria and other cerebellar signs.

Patients with dystonia often have tremor in the dystonic limb. However, in contrast to other types of tremor, it is usually irregular and non-rhythmic.

All these types of tremor occur in the context of other diseases and are rare. Most cases of isolated tremor are due to a monosymptomatic disorder known as essential tremor.

Essential tremor
Essential tremor is the most common movement disorder and is seen in 5-7% of people aged 65 years or more. The aetiology and pathogenesis of essential tremor are not fully understood. However, the findings of postmortem examinations and functional neuro-imaging studies suggest involvement of the cerebellum, the inferior olive, the red nucleus and the thalamus. The evidence also suggests that dysfunction of GABA (gamma aminobutyric acid) neurotransmission plays an important role in the pathogenesis of essential tremor. The disease tends to run in families, but the contribution of genetic factors is not known.

Different criteria are used for the diagnosis of essential tremor. Generally, a confident diagnosis can be made in the presence of a positive family history; a normal neurological examination (except the tremor); and moderately severe, bilateral tremor of at least one limb. The tremor must be postural, kinetic or both. (The kinetic component should be present in at least four tasks, e.g. drinking water with a spoon, performance of the finger–nose test, drawing a spiral, eating.) In addition, other causes of tremor, including excessive alcohol consumption, Parkinson's disease, hyperthyroidism, drugs, etc., should be excluded. Typically, essential tremor is increased by anxiety, stress and caffeine, and decreased by alcohol.

Treatment should be considered when the tremor causes functional disability. Primidone or propranolol are usually effective first-line drugs. Second choice drugs include gabapentin and topiramate. Deep brain stimulation of the thalamus is used in severe cases refractory to medical treatment.

Parkinson's disease

Parkinson's disease (PD), also called paralysis agitans or idiopathic parkinsonism, is a common neurodegenerative disorder. It is estimated that 2 adults out of every 1000 develop the disease every year. The prevalence of PD is 10-15 times its incidence rate. PD is predominantly a disease of older people. However, in approximately 10% of cases the disease occurs before the age of 45 years. It is more common in males.

Pathology

PD is caused by the degeneration of the pigmented substantia nigra neurons resulting in deficiency of dopamine. The neurons contain an eosinophilic protein known as Lewy bodies. Usually, more than 80% of the dopaminergic nigral neurons die before the patient develops significant symptoms. Neuronal loss also occurs in the brain stem, but it is less extensive than in the substantia nigra.

Clinical features

The onset of PD is insidious and its course is slowly progressive. Typically, in the early stage of the disease the symptoms are either ignored by the patient or are attributed to old age. The core features of PD are bradykinesia, tremor, muscle rigidity, gait disturbances and impairment of the postural reflexes. The disease always starts on one side of the body and spreads to the other side after a few years.

Bradykinesia is defined as the slow initiation and execution of voluntary movements. The time to carry out everyday activities, such as personal care, writing, eating, etc., becomes longer as the disease progresses. Initially the difficulties occur with fine movements, but eventually all motor activities are affected.

Rigidity is increase in muscle tone. Typically, when the muscle tone is assessed by flexing and extending a limb, the examiner feels resistance which gives way briefly and then it is felt again. This phenomenon is often described as cogwheel rigidity. In advanced disease, rigidity of the axial muscles results in trunk flexion and a stooped posture. The combination of bradykinesia and rigidity explains many other features of parkinsonism, e.g. reduced rate of blinking, reduced facial expression (hypomimia), micrographia, and drooling of saliva due to slow swallowing.

Tremor is observed in a third of patients with PD. Usually it affects one hand and is present at rest (rest tremor), but occasionally it is triggered by a voluntary movement (action tremor). Typically, the thumb beats against the index finger. The tremor is increased by anxiety and is absent during sleep. Some patients develop mouth tremor or tremor in the lower limb.

In the early stages of PD, the gait abnormalities consist of a reduced swing of the arm on the affected side and shortening of the stride length. As the disease progresses, the patient starts to shuffle and he becomes unable to move from time to time. These 'freezing episodes' usually occur when the patient tries to turn around or walk through doorways. Poor balance and frequent falls are common at this stage of the disease. A contributing factor to this is the impairment of postural reflexes. Constipation, orthostatic hypotension, dysarthria and dysphonia are also features of advanced PD.

Differential diagnosis

PD should be distinguished from symptomatic parkinsonism and from a group of disorders known as the Parkinson-plus syndromes.

The most common cause of symptomatic parkinsonism is neuroleptic drugs. Other causes include encephalitis, cerebrovascular disease and toxins, e.g. carbon monoxide, manganese and mercury. The medical history, the rapid onset and the simultaneous involvement of both sides of the body help to differentiate symptomatic parkinsonism from PD.

The Parkinson-plus Syndromes (PPS) are a group of rare degenerative disorders that include multisystem atrophy and progressive supranuclear palsy. Patients with these disorders present with features similar to those of PD and, in addition, they exhibit other neurological signs such as pyramidal tract, eye signs or severe failure of the autonomic nervous system. Other features of the PPS are rapid disease progression, onset before the age of 40, bilateral signs on first presentation and poor response to adequate doses of levodopa.

Treatment

The main drugs that are used for the treatment of PD are levodopa and the dopamine agonists. Anticholinergic drugs, such as benzhexol and orphenadrine, are not very effective and often result in unacceptable adverse effects. Amantadine stimulates the release of dopamine from the surviving substantia nigra neurons and is most useful in the early stages of the disease, but its beneficial effect usually does not last more than a few weeks.

Treatment should only be started when PD causes significant functional disability. The drug of first choice is either a dopamine agonist, or a combination of levodopa and a dopa-decarboxylase inhibitor, such as carbidopa or benserazide. (The dopa-decarboxylase inhibitor reduces the breakdown of dopamine in the gut.) Because high doses of these drugs often cause serious psychiatric adverse effects and postural hypotension, the smallest effective dose should be used and maintained for the longest possible period. The addition of a type B monoamine oxidase inhibitor, e.g. selegiline, to levodopa improves the control of symptoms and usually allows the dose of levodopa to be reduced by a third. The catechol-O-methyltransferase inhibitors entacapone and tolcapone may also be used together with levodopa in advanced disease, but they may cause serious liver toxicity.

Pramipexole, ropinirole and rotigotine are the most frequently used oral dopamine agonists. They are effective when used alone in the early stages of PD and when combined with levodopa in advanced disease. Apomorphine is the only injectable dopamine agonist available at present and is usually used when other drug regimens fail.

The treatment of PD should be individualised to fit the patient's lifestyle. In the early stages of the disease it is usually sufficient to administer the drugs every 6 or 8 hours. However, more frequent doses (every 2 or 3 hours) are usually required as the disease progresses because the number of surviving dopaminergic neurons and the brain's storage capacity of exogenous dopamine fall. Small frequent doses reduce the dyskinesia, which is a common adverse effect of levodopa and dopamine agonists, and improve the control of the symptoms of PD.

Surgery may be considered in the treatment of patients with severe symptoms that are refractory to drug therapy. Various procedures, including pallidotomy and deep brain stimulation, have been used.

Prognosis

The course of PD is invariably progressive, but the rate of clinical deterioration varies between individuals. Most patients develop significant disability 15-20 years after diagnosis, and 1 in 3 patients develop dementia. Life expectancy is also shortened by PD. The most common cause of death is aspiration pneumonia.

Dystonia

Dystonia is the sustained or intermittent involuntary contraction of a group of muscles resulting in abnormal movements or postures. The dystonia can affect any skeletal muscle and may be generalised or localised.

Dystonia is classified into primary (idiopathic) or secondary (symptomatic) dystonia. The exact cause of primary dystonia is not known, but genetic factors, at least in some cases, appear to be important. To date, more than 20 'dystonia genes' have been identified. Mutation of these genes has been found in some patients with early- and late-onset dystonia. The mode of inheritance in the majority of cases is autosomal dominant with low penetrance, but autosomal recessive transmission also occurs. However, no dystonia gene has been found in some familial cases. Secondary dystonia may result from treatment with various drugs, such as neuroleptic drugs and metoclopramide. Other causes of secondary dystonia include anoxic brain injury, cerebrovascular disease and encephalitis.

The pathogenesis of dystonia is not fully understood. No structural changes in the basal ganglia have been found in primary dystonia. However, functional magnetic resonance scans and positron emission tomography have demonstrated an imbalance between the neurotransmitters acetylcholine, dopamine and gamma aminobutyric acid (GABA) in the basal ganglia and prefrontal cortex.

Cervical dystonia

Cervical dystonia, also known as spasmodic torticollis, is the most common form of localised dystonia. There is a large variation in its reported incidence and prevalence. Between 8 and 12 adults per one million of the population develop cervical dystonia every year, and at any one time there are 28 to 183 per one million who suffer from it. The disease is twice as common in females as in males. In most patients the onset of cervical dystonia is between the age of 40 and 50 years.

Clinical features

The onset of cervical dystonia is gradual and its course is slowly progressive. The most common symptoms on presentation are abnormal head postures and severe, constant neck pain. The latter occurs in 75% of cases. As shown in figure 7.1 below, any one of four head postures may be present. The head is either tilted forward (antecollis), backward (retrocollis), towards the shoulder (laterocollis), or turned to left or right (rotational torticollis). In some patients a combination of head postures is also seen. In chronic dystonia the affected neck muscle hypertrophy.

In addition to neck pain and the involuntary contraction of neck muscles, other symptoms and signs are often present. More than a third of patients report mild to moderately severe dysphagia. Depression is common. An irregular head tremor, dysarthria and tenderness, and elevation of the shoulder muscles are sometimes present. The symptoms of dystonia are sometimes alleviated by touching the neck muscles. However, the effect of these 'sensory tricks' is usually transient. Stress is known to aggravate the dystonia.

Figure 7.1
The different head postures in cervical dystonia

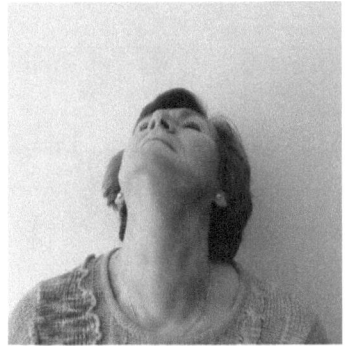

Retrocollis

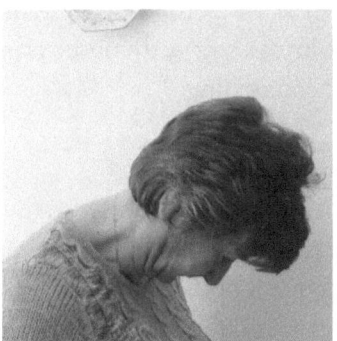

Antecollis

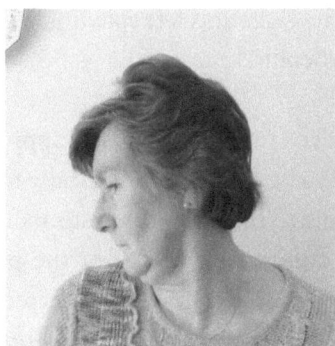

Laterocollis

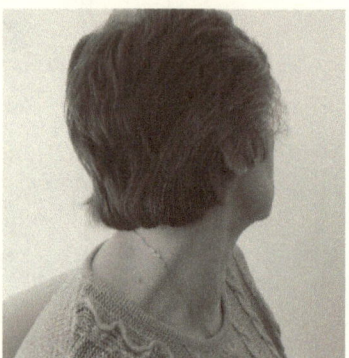

Rotational Torticollis

The diagnosis of cervical dystonia is mainly based on the patient's symptoms and clinical examination. Investigations are of limited value except for the exclusion of the secondary dystonias. Genetic tests yield positive results mostly in cases of early onset primary dystonia and are essential before genetic counselling.

Treatment and prognosis
There is no cure for cervical dystonia. However, the symptoms can be very well controlled in most patients, especially in the early stage of the disease. The treatment of first choice is botulinum toxin injections into the affected neck muscles. The selection of muscles for the toxin injection depends on the classification of the dystonia. For example, in rotational torticollis the ipsilateral sternomastoid and the contralateral splenius capitis muscles are injected. By contrast, the right and left splenius capitis muscles should be injected in cases of retrocollis.

The beneficial effect of the toxin usually lasts approximately four months and the injections need to be repeated periodically to maintain the optimal control of the symptoms. In cases of dystonia refractory to medical treatment, deep brain stimulation (DBS) of the pallidum (implantation into the pallidum of electric electrodes connected to an external pulse generator) may be considered. Selective surgical resection of the dystonic muscles is another treatment option.

In the past various drugs, including anticholinergic medication, baclofen, the benzodiazepines and clonazepam, have been used for the treatment of cervical dystonia. However, these drugs are usually ineffective and frequently result in severe adverse effects. Similarly, stereotactic surgery of the thalamus carries considerable risk and its results cannot be accurately predicted.

The prognosis of cervical dystonia is influenced by the disease severity and the patient's age at the time of disease onset. It is best in young patients and when the disease is mild. These patients usually have long remissions. Spontaneous recovery from cervical dystonia has been reported, but it appears to be very rare.

Huntington's disease

Huntington's disease (HD) is a basal ganglia disorder characterised by abnormal movements, cognitive impairment and psychiatric symptoms. The disease is genetically determined and results from a gene mutation on chromosome 4. The mode of inheritance is autosomal dominant. In approximately 5% of cases, there is no family history of HD; this can be accounted for by spontaneous mutations or illegitimacy. The prevalence of HD varies according to ethnicity. In Caucasians the prevalence is 5-6 cases per 100,000 of the population. By contrast, it is less than 1 in 100,000 in Asian populations.

Pathology

The main pathological changes in Huntington's disease (HD) occur in the striatum and, to a lesser extent, in the cerebral cortex. Significant atrophy of the head of the caudate nucleus and putamen precedes the clinical manifestations of the disease by 12-15 years. The number of dopamine receptors in the striatum is reduced, but there is an increased receptor sensitivity to dopamine in the early stage of the disease. The substantia nigra is relatively spared, except in juvenile HD. In the late stages of the disease, dopamine deficiency develops and corresponds to the hypokinetic-rigid phase of advanced HD.

Cortical atrophy of the temporo-frontal region also occurs early. Severe atrophy of the frontal cortex is particularly common in patients with the hypokinetic-rigid form of HD.

Clinical features

In most cases, the first clinical manifestations of HD are usually in the fifth decade of life. In approximately 5-10% of patients the disease onset is before the age of 20 years (Juvenile HD, or Westphal variant of HD).

In the early phase of HD, most patients present with hyperkinetic abnormal movements, usually chorea. Dystonia, athetosis and tremor are other manifestations of the disease. As the disease advances, these involuntary movements are replaced by a hypokinetic-rigid state similar to that of Parkinson's disease. In Juvenile HD, patients present with the hypokinetic-rigid form of the disease from the start.

The psychiatric symptoms of HD are many. Personality change is common. The patient may become irritable, impulsive or aggressive. Anxiety and depression frequently occur in the early phase of the disease, and an estimated one in four patients attempts suicide. Some patients also develop psychosis.

Cognitive decline may precede, follow or develop simultaneously with the motor symptoms. It is relentlessly progressive and culminates in overt dementia.

A genetic DNA test is available for the confirmation of the diagnosis in symptomatic patients and for the detection of family members who are at risk of developing the disease. Genetic counselling should always be offered before the genetic test.

Treatment and prognosis

There is no cure for Huntington's disease. The management consists of the treatment of the symptoms and the practical and emotional support for the patients and their families.

Tetrabenazine is very effective for the control of chorea. The dose should be titrated up gradually in increments of 12.5 mg until the symptom is controlled. The maximum daily dose is 100 mg. Amantadine (300 mg/day) and riluzole (200 mg/day) are other alternatives. Botulinum toxin injections are indicated when disabling focal dystonia is present, and anti-parkinsonian drugs are useful in the late stages of HD and in Juvenile HD.

Specific psychiatric treatment for depression, anxiety and psychosis is indicated in most cases. Behavioural therapy is usually beneficial only in the early stages of the disease.

The course of HD is slowly progressive and death usually occurs 15-20 years after the initial diagnosis.

Blepharospasm

Idiopathic blepharospasm (IB) is a rare focal dystonia of unknown cause. It is more common in females and usually starts in late middle life. The main underlying abnormality in IB is an involuntary contraction of the orbicularis oculi muscle, relaxation of the levator palpebrae superiors and upward deviation of the eyeball.

Clinical features

The onset of IB is gradual and its course is often progressive. After a few years, most patients with IB develop other forms of focal or segmental dystonias, or spasmodic torticollis. In the early stages of the disease, patients usually experience mild intermittent eye symptoms such as dryness, photosensitivity or increased frequency of blinking. The diagnosis is usually obvious when the patients start to experience intermittent voluntary closure of both eyes usually lasting 15-30 seconds. The attacks occur with variable frequency and may be precipitated by bright light, walking, reading and emotional stress.

Differential diagnosis

IB should be distinguished from the voluntary eyelid closure that is often observed in patients with photophobia due to eye disease. A variety of drugs, e.g. neuroleptics, lithium and lamotrigine, may cause blepharospasm. Other differential diagnoses include habit tics and blepharospasm associated with Parkinson's disease.

Treatment

Partial or complete spontaneous remission occurs in a minority of patients, especially in the first five years of the disease. The treatment of first choice is botulinum toxin injections into the orbicularis oculi muscle. Surgical resection of the protractor muscle of the eyelid or avulsion of the facial nerve may be considered when botulinum toxin is contraindicated or is ineffective.

CHAPTER 8

DEMYELINATING DISEASES

Demyelination of the CNS may result from inflammation, metabolic disorders (e.g. the rapid correction of hyponatraemia), ischaemic-hypoxic brain injury, or following viral infections, such as measles, mumps, chickenpox and infectious mononucleosis.

Demyelination is the destruction of the myelin sheath of the axons. The myelin sheath is a lipid-rich membrane wrapped around the axon. The sheath is not continuous. Areas that are not covered by myelin occur at regular intervals along the axon. These areas are known as the nodes of Ranvier. The myelin sheath insulates the axon and facilitates the fast transmission of the nerve impulse from one node of Ranvier to the next, a process known as saltatory conduction. Therefore, demyelination blocks nerve conduction. Another function of the myelin sheath is that it provides trophic support for the axon. Consequently, demyelination also leads to secondary axonal degeneration. The most common cause of demyelination is multiple sclerosis (also called disseminated sclerosis).

Multiple sclerosis

Multiple sclerosis (MS) is an immune-mediated inflammatory disorder of the CNS. The cause of the disease is not known. However, genetic predisposition and environmental factors appear to be important. Although MS is not hereditary, certain genetic variations, e.g. the histocompatibility antigens DR15 and DQ6, increase the risk of developing the disease.

The importance of environmental factors in developing MS is suggested by migration studies. For example, adults who migrate from a high risk to a low risk area retain the high risk of their birthplace. The opposite is also true. It is thought that an, as yet unidentified, infective agent that is acquired in childhood but remains latent triggers the onset of MS later in life. Epidemiological studies have also shown that cigarette smoking increases the risk of MS, while high levels of vitamin D have a protective effect.

MS is very common, but there is a wide variation between different parts of the world in its incidence and prevalence. The disease is more common in Nordic countries, Scotland and Canada than in any other part of Europe or North America. It is rare in Africa and South America. Recent studies have also shown a significant increase in the occurrence of MS worldwide. Although this may be due to improved access to healthcare and better diagnosis, changes in lifestyle, longer life expectancy and other factors could also be important. MS is more common in females and its onset is usually between the ages of 20-30 years. It is very rare in children.

Pathology

There are four distinct clinicopathological types of MS: classical MS, neuromyelitis optica (Devic's disease), acute fulminant MS (Marburg type), and concentric MS (Balo's sclerosis). The last two types are very rare. The pathological changes and clinical course of acute fulminant MS are similar to those of severe acute disseminated encephalomyelitis. The histopathological abnormalities in concentric MS consist of concentric rings of intact fibres within an area of demyelinated tissue. Its clinical course, in most cases, resembles primary progressive MS.

The histological examination of the acute lesion of MS shows destruction of the myelin sheath with relative sparing of the axon, and infiltration of lymphocytes and mononuclear cells in perivascular areas. In the chronic phase of the disease there is axonal degeneration, grey matter inflammatory lesions and neuronal degeneration in the cerebral cortex, and meningeal inflammation in addition to the demyelination. Partial spontaneous remyelination occurs during the remissions of MS. The areas of demyelination (called plaques) vary in size and are randomly distributed. In chronic disease, brain atrophy is common. Although the histopathological changes described above are the hallmark of MS, the acute lesions evolve differently in different subgroups of patients. This suggests that more than one mechanism is probably involved in the pathogenesis of MS.

Demyelination in classical MS occurs mostly in the visual pathways, periventricular white matter, the brain stem, the cerebellum, the cervical and thoracic segments of the spinal cord, and the cerebral cortex, especially the frontal and temporal lobes.

Clinical classification of classical MS

MS is classified according to its clinical course into relapsing-remitting, secondary progressive and primary progressive MS. The relapsing-remitting form of MS is more common in females and occurs usually between the ages of 20 and 30 years. By contrast, primary progressive MS occurs with equal frequency in males and females and tends to develop later in life.

Relapsing-remitting MS is characterised by acute episodes of neurological deficits, e.g. optic neuritis, followed by complete or partial recovery. This form of the disease accounts for 85% of all cases of MS. Secondary progressive MS usually develops 5-15 years after the onset of the relapsing-remitting form. In primary progressive MS, there are no clear-cut remissions from the initial onset of the disease and the neurological deterioration is progressive for at least a year or more. Approximately 15% of patients with MS have the primary progressive disease.

Clinical features

The onset of MS is often preceded by an infection, a stressful life event or physical injury. Patients may present with any combination of symptoms and signs of damage to the motor or the sensory systems, cerebellum, brain stem or cerebral cortex. However, the initial presentation is frequently with unilateral optic neuritis or transverse myelitis. Trigeminal neuralgia, fatigue, seizures, depression and other psychiatric symptoms are also common. Cognitive impairment is usually a feature of advanced disease. In the relapsing and remitting form of MS, the neurological deficits resolve after a few weeks either partially or completely. The remission may last months or years and is followed by the emergence of new symptoms. After each such cycle there is usually a certain degree of residual permanent disability.

Diagnosis

The diagnosis of MS is made by demonstrating, from the history and findings of the neurological examination, the presence of at least two demyelinating lesions in separate anatomical regions and that the lesions have occurred at different times. The provisional clinical diagnosis is confirmed with evidence from laboratory tests and brain imaging.

The inflammatory nature of MS is demonstrated with CSF analysis. CSF examination shows a moderate (50-100 cells per mm^3) lymphocytic pleocytosis and raised protein (usually less than 1 g/L). Oligoclonal bands are also present on CSF electrophoresis.

Delay in the visual evoked or sensory evoked responses confirms involvement of the visual or sensory pathways, respectively.

MRI brain and spinal cord scans are invaluable in the diagnosis of MS. They can demonstrate the presence of lesions in different anatomical regions (dissemination in space), as well as the simultaneous presence of multifocal chronic plaques and new inflammatory changes (dissemination in time).

Differential diagnosis

The early diagnosis of MS is often difficult because typically the initial presentation is with a single episode of neurological symptoms. The term 'clinically isolated syndrome' (CIS) is used to describe this clinical presentation.

The CIS should be distinguished from non-MS monophasic demyelinating diseases, such as acute disseminated encephalomyelitis. The differential diagnosis also includes infectious diseases (syphilis, Lyme disease, HIV, cytomegalovirus infection), nutritional deficiencies (B12 deficiency), cerebrovascular disease (lacunar infarcts), inflammatory disorders (sarcoidosis) and metabolic abnormalities (rapid correction of hyponatraemia).

Treatment

The aim of treatment of MS is to minimise the neurological deficits by treating the initial acute episode or relapse, to control the distressing symptoms of the disease, to prevent or minimise the functional disability, and to reduce the risk of future relapses.

Methyl prednisolone (0.5 g daily for 5 days by mouth, or 1 g intravenously daily for 5 days) is the treatment of choice for an acute relapse. Plasma exchange may be considered for severe fulminant cases and when the response to methyl prednisolone is poor.

A coordinated supportive care, rehabilitation and the control of the distressing symptoms of MS, e.g. spasticity, depression, emotional lability, incontinence, etc., are an important part of the long-term management of MS.

Patients with relapsing-remitting MS also benefit from disease-modifying drugs. These drugs reduce the frequency and severity of relapses, and also delay brain atrophy and functional disability. Many disease-modifying drugs are available and include interferon beta, glatiramer, dimethyl fumarate, natalizumab, and others. Treatment with these drugs should be initiated by a specialist.

Other demyelinating diseases

Acute disseminated encephalomyelitis (ADEM)

ADEM is a self-limiting, acute inflammatory demyelinating disease of the CNS. The disease is usually monophasic, but relapses occur in 5-10% of patients. In contrast to MS, the inflammatory changes of ADEM are severe, but the demyelination is not extensive. ADEM is most common in children and usually follows childhood viral infections or vaccination. The clinical presentation is with headaches, systemic symptoms, seizures and focal neurological signs. Stupor and coma often develop quickly. Brain imaging demonstrates widespread usually symmetrical lesions. There are usually mild non-specific changes on CSF analysis. Treatment is with high doses of corticosteroids. Complete recovery occurs in approximately 80% of cases.

Neuromyelitis optica (Devic's disease)

Neuromyelitis optica is an inflammatory disorder characterised by bilateral optic neuritis and transverse myelitis that occur simultaneously, and the presence of specific antibodies in the serum (AQP4-IgG antibodies). In recent years, the term 'Neuromyelitis Optica Spectrum Disorders' (NMOSD) has been adopted to incorporate disorders in which cortical and brain stem lesions are present in addition to bilateral optic neuritis and transverse myelitis. AQP4-IgG antibodies may or may not be present. Some patients develop unexplained hiccups, nausea and vomiting. The CSF contains a large number of polymorphonuclear leucocytes. Typically, there are no oligoclonal bands in the CSF.

Progressive multifocal leukoencephalopathy (PML)

PML is an acute rapidly progressive demyelinating disease caused by a polyoma virus (papovavirus) known as JC virus (John Cunningham virus). The disease occurs in patients with severely depressed cell immunity, e.g. HIV/AIDS, lymphoma, and is characterised by widespread CNS demyelination. The patient presents with headaches; seizures; ataxia; motor, sensory and visual symptoms; and cognitive impairment.

Brain imaging (preferably MRI scan) shows multiple small white matter lesions. The diagnosis is confirmed by identifying the JC virus DNA with the polymerase chain reaction (PCR) test. Treatment is with plasma exchange and supportive therapy. The mortality rate is high.

CHAPTER 9

THE NEURODEGENERATIVE DISORDERS

Degeneration is the premature and pathological deterioration in the cellular and tissue structure and function. Degenerative disorders of the nervous system are characterised by the destruction of the neurons and myelin sheath with subsequent phagocytosis and gliosis. Neuronal degeneration should be distinguished from neuronal atrophy. The latter is a predictable physiological and age-related process that is not due to disease. Atrophic neurons are small in size but otherwise morphologically normal.

The mechanisms of neurodegeneration are not fully understood. However, there is evidence that the excessive production of peroxides and free radicals (oxidative stress), defective DNA repair and the accumulation of abnormal proteins in the neuron are implicated in the pathogenesis of the neurodegenerative diseases. In addition, genetic mutations and environmental factors influence the development and course of these disorders.

The characteristic features of the neurodegenerative disorders
Neurodegenerative diseases have a number of features in common. Each neurodegenerative disease selectively affects a specific group of neurons, e.g. degeneration of the motor nuclei and their axons occurs in motor neurone disease, whereas degeneration of substantia nigra pars compacta cells causes Parkinson's disease. Typically, the neuronal degeneration starts many years before the first manifestations of the disease and the clinical signs appear only after the degeneration of a critical number of neurons. The neurological signs are always bilateral and are often symmetrical. The disease onset is gradual and its course, in the vast majority of cases, is slowly progressive and usually spans a decade or more.

The most common neurodegenerative diseases are dementia, Parkinson's disease and related disorders, Huntington's disease, motor neurone disease, and the cerebellar ataxias.

Dementia

Dementia is a disease characterised by progressive global cognitive decline, personality change and psychiatric symptoms. In most cases the disease onset is after the age of 64 years (senile dementia), but young-onset (presenile) dementia (usually defined as dementia in the age group 45-64 years) is not uncommon. Primary young-onset dementia is often a late manifestation of rare childhood neurodegenerative hereditary disorders, such as Gaucher's disease. A common cause of early onset dementia is Down's syndrome.

Down's syndrome

Down's syndrome is the most common cause of congenital learning disability. It is due to a chromosomal abnormality (an extra copy of chromosome 21) and its incidence is influenced by maternal age. (The older the mother at the time of gestation, the higher the risk of having a baby with Down's syndrome.) In addition to the intellectual disability, there are typical craniofacial abnormalities, such as a small chin, slanted eyes, flat nasal bridge and a small mouth. Congenital heart disease (atrial and ventricular septal defects) and gastrointestinal abnormalities (duodenal stenosis, megacolon) are common. Dementia occurs in 70% of patients by the age of 30-40 years.

Dementia due to systemic disease

Although dementia most frequently results from a primary neurodegenerative disorder, it is sometimes a complication of systemic disease. Cerebrovascular disease is the most common cause of dementia due to systemic disorders (see Chapter 4). Postmortem studies have shown that vascular dementia and Alzheimer's disease frequently coexist in the same patient. Other causes of dementia include infections (e.g. HIV infection, syphilis, chronic tuberculous or fungal meningitis), inflammatory disorders (e.g. multiple sclerosis, neurosarcoidosis), toxic substances (e.g. alcohol abuse), metabolic disorders (e.g. renal or hepatic failure), and chronic traumatic encephalopathy due to repeated (usually mild) brain injury.

The clinical features of dementia

As a rule of thumb, the onset of dementia is gradual. However, in some cases the symptoms may be precipitated suddenly by an acute illness. As described in the following sections, the initial clinical presentation depends on the subtype of dementia. In young-onset dementia psychiatric symptoms often predominate. By contrast, memory impairment is usually an early symptom of dementia developing in old age. With disease progression, a combination of global cognitive impairment and personality change become evident. Memory, reasoning, judgement and emotional responses are affected. Clinical examination reveals language abnormalities, visual-spatial disorientation, apraxia and agnosia. Marked deterioration in social skills, disinhibition, hallucinations, delusions, paranoia, immobility and mutism are late features of the disease.

Dementia is classified according to the location of most of the pathological changes, i.e. whether most of the degeneration is in the cortex or subcortical structures, and by its clinical features into cortical and subcortical dementia. Patients with cortical dementia typically have significant memory impairment and focal frontal, temporal and occipital lobe signs, e.g. dysphasia, dyspraxia and agnosia. By contrast, the main features of subcortical dementia are slow cognitive processing, personality change, apathy, depression and mild extrapyramidal signs.

The diagnosis of dementia

The diagnosis of dementia is based on the clinical symptoms and signs, and is confirmed with a formal assessment of cognitive function, for example, the Mini-Mental State Examination (MMSE) or similar psychometric tests.

The MMSE test is simple, reliable and easy to use. It is a standardised scale consisting of 8 subscales that contain a total of 30 items. It tests orientation, memory, recall, attention, calculation, repetition and the ability to follow complex commands. Each item correctly answered is awarded 1 point. A score that is less than 24 points indicates cognitive impairment. The items of the MMSE test and their scores are listed in table 9.1.

Table 9.1
The MMES:

Item	Questions	Score
Orientation in time	What is the year, season, date, day, time?	5
Orientation in place	Where are we now? State, county, town, hospital, floor.	5
Registration	Name 3 unrelated objects and ask the patient to repeat them.	3
Attention and calculation	Serially subtract 7 from 100.	5
Recall	Ask the patient to name the 3 objects which he repeated earlier.	3
Language	Ask the patient to name 2 simple objects (watch, pen).	2
Repetition	Ask patient to repeat the sentence 'no ifs, ands, or buts'.	1
Complex commands	1. Hand the patient a piece of paper and ask him to take in his right hand, fold it and put back on the floor.	3
	2. Ask the patient to write a short sentence containing a verb and a noun.	2
	3. Draw 2 interlocking pentagons and ask the patient to copy them.	1

Once the diagnosis of dementia is made, its cause should be established. Dementia due to systemic disease should be distinguished from the dementias of primary neurodegenerative disease. The medical history and clinical examination are often helpful. For example, a history of diabetes, hypertension and other stroke risk factors is a clue to a vascular aetiology. In addition, cognitive deterioration often occurs suddenly in vascular dementia and after a few weeks the cognitive function usually improves, but then suddenly deteriorates again. This cyclical pattern of deterioration-improvement- deterioration is usually repeated several times.

Brain imaging and laboratory tests are essential for the differential diagnosis in all cases of dementia. Screening should include a full blood count; liver, renal and thyroid function tests; blood glucose; serum cholesterol; and serological tests for syphilis. Other tests may be indicated depending on the medical history and findings of the clinical examination.

Dementia due to neurodegenerative disease
Alzheimer's disease, frontotemporal dementia and Lewy body dementia are the most common dementias due to neurodegenerative disease. They differ from each other by the type of abnormal protein that accumulates in the neurons, the part of the cortex that is preferentially most affected and by some of their early clinical manifestations (table 9.2).

Alzheimer's disease

Alzheimer's disease (AD) is the most common type of dementia. It accounts for approximately a third of all cases of early onset dementia and for around 70-75% of the dementias occurring after the age of 64 years. The incidence and prevalence of the disease increase with age. An estimated 10% of 65-year-old men and women and more than a third of those who are 85 years old have AD. In most cases the disease is sporadic, but there is also a rare familial form with an autosomal dominant mode of inheritance. The mutation of three different genes has been implicated in the pathogenesis of late-onset (sporadic) AD. They are thought to increase the risk of developing dementia by interacting with environmental factors, such as abnormal lipid metabolism and dysfunction of the immune system.

The pathological changes in AD consist of diffuse cerebral atrophy, vacuolar degeneration of cortical neurons, astrocytic proliferation, senile plaques (accumulation of amyloid and dystrophic axons and dendrites) and neurofibrillary tangles (intra cellular deposits of tau protein). Synaptic function is disrupted due to abnormalities of acetylcholine and gamma aminobutyric acid (GABA) neurotransmission.

Treatment of AD with acetylcholinesterase inhibitors and memantine is effective in the early phase of the disease. Either donepezil (5-10 mg once daily), galantamine (8-24 mg/day), rivastigmine (1.5-6 mg/day) or memantine (5-20 mg/day) may be used. Treatment should be started with a small dose and the dose gradually increased over several weeks. In addition to drug therapy, cognitive rehabilitation is effective in the early phase of the disease. As with all subtypes of dementia, there is no effective treatment in the advanced stage. The management consists of the control of symptoms, and the practical and emotional support of the patient, his family and carers.

Frontotemporal dementia

Frontotemporal dementia (FTD) is the third most common type of dementia after AD and vascular dementia. It has a prevalence of 15-22 cases per 100,000 of the population in Europe and North America. FTD is a familial disorder with an autosomal dominant mode of inheritance and 100% penetrance. The onset is usually in middle age or earlier.

In contrast to AD and other types of dementia, the degenerative changes occur mainly in the frontal and temporal lobes, and relatively spare other parts of the cortex and subcortical structures. The intracellular accumulation of tau protein (not amyloid as in AD) and the early clinical symptoms also distinguish FTD from AD.

In the early phase of FTD, patients usually present with behavioural symptoms and progressive non-fluent dysphasia. The early behavioural symptoms often resemble psychiatric disorders. Depression, indifference, socially unacceptable conduct and impulsivity often precede other clinical features of the disease. Anomia, agrammatism, and sparse repetitive speech are also early signs. The language impairment gradually becomes more severe and progresses to mutism. Pyramidal tract signs are also common. Advanced FTD is clinically indistinguishable from other forms of dementia. There is no effective treatment and the disease shortens life expectancy. The median survival after diagnosis is 5 to 12 years.

Lewy body dementia

Lewy body dementia (LBD) accounts for approximately 5% of all dementias. The disease is usually sporadic, but a familial form due to the mutation of the alpha-synuclein gene has also been reported. The pathological changes in LBD involve the cortex and the basal ganglia, and are characterised by the deposition of Lewy bodies (eosinophilic cytoplasmic structures made of two proteins: alpha-synuclein and ubiquitin).

The main early features of LBD are global and progressive cognitive impairment, parkinsonism, visual hallucinations and fluctuating cognition, and alertness. Typically, the cognitive decline precedes the symptoms of parkinsonism by at least a year, but the two may develop concurrently. This distinguishes LBD from Parkinson's disease dementia (which follows the symptoms of parkinsonism by many years). In contrast to AD, the cognitive deficits in the early phase of LBD are typical of subcortical dementia and consist of reduced attention and disruption of the frontal lobe executive function, rather than memory impairment. Poor judgement, apathy, disinhibition and depressed mood are early signs. In the later stages of the disease the symptoms resemble those of other types of dementia.

There are no specific clinical tests for the diagnosis of LBD. Dilatation of the cerebral ventricles, and reduced size of the hippocampus and putamen are the typical findings on MRI scans.

Treatment with small doses of L-dopa may improve the motor manifestations of the disease. Symptomatic treatment of depression and psychosis is sometimes necessary. In advanced disease most patients require institutional care.

Table 9.2
Summary of the distinguishing features of the neurodegenerative dementias:

Dementia subtype	Abnormal neuronal protein	Part of the brain that is most affected	Distinguishing early clinical features
Alzheimer's disease	Amyloid	Diffuse	Memory impairment
Frontotemporal dementia	Tau protein	Frontal and temporal lobes	Behavioural symptoms, non-fluent dysphasia
Lewy body dementia	Synuclein and ubiquitin	Subcortical structures	Parkinsonism, hallucinations, fluctuating alertness

The hereditary cerebellar ataxias

The hereditary cerebellar ataxias is a diverse group of genetically-determined degenerative disorders with an onset usually in childhood. Onset of these disorders in adult life is rare. The mode of inheritance is either autosomal recessive or autosomal dominant. Cerebellar degeneration is a common feature in all cases, and the course of the disease is progressive and invariably results in significant disability by middle age, or earlier.

The autosomal recessive ataxias
More than 20 different types of the autosomal recessive ataxias have been identified. The most common is Friedreich's ataxia.

Friedreich's ataxia
Friedreich's ataxia accounts for 50% of all the autosomal recessive ataxias. The onset is in childhood, but there is also a rare adult onset type. Pathologically, the disease is characterised by degeneration of the cerebellum, the posterior columns of the spinal cord, the cuneate and gracile nuclei, the dorsal root ganglia, the pyramidal tracts and peripheral nerves.

The clinical features of the disease are ataxia and other cerebellar signs (described in Chapter 1), severe sensory neuropathy, proprioceptive sensory loss and upper motor neuron signs. Skeletal abnormalities, e.g. scoliosis and pes cavus, diabetes mellitus and cardiomyopathy are common.

The disability caused by Friedreich's ataxia is progressive. Most children are wheelchair dependent by the age of 15 years. Life expectancy is usually shortened to 40-50 years.

The autosomal dominant ataxias

The autosomal dominant ataxias are called the spinocerebellar ataxias (SCA). To date more than 30 types of SCA have been identified. Cerebellar symptoms and signs are present in all types. In addition, signs of brain stem, pyramidal or extra pyramidal tracts involvement, ophthalmoplegia, peripheral neuropathies, dementia and epileptic seizures occur in various combinations depending on the type of the SCA.

The hereditary ataxias should be distinguished from ataxias acquired in childhood. These may be due to viral infections, stroke, hypoxic encephalopathy, trauma, immune dysfunction, nutritional deficiencies, toxic agents (e.g. organic solvents) or a non-metastatic manifestation of malignancy (i.e. paraneoplastic).

The diagnosis is based on the family history, the clinical presentation, and course of the disease and clinical investigations, including brain imaging and genetic testing.

There is no specific treatment for the hereditary ataxias. The management consists of the treatment of the co-morbidities, e.g. diabetes and cardiomyopathy in Friedreich's ataxia, interventions to reduce the functional disability due to the ataxia (for details see the relevant section of Chapter 2), rehabilitation and supportive care.

Motor neurone disease

Motor neurone disease (MND) is a degenerative disorder of the motor system. The incidence of new cases of MND in Europe is approximately 1 case per 100,000 of the population per year. The prevalence is 4-5 patients per 100,000 of the population. In most cases the disease is diagnosed in the fourth or fifth decade of life. Most cases are sporadic, but MND is a familial hereditary disorder in 5-10% of patients. It is thought that the degenerative changes in sporadic MND result from a combination of genetic predisposition and environmental factors. Patients with MND have clinicopathological features that resemble those of frontotemporal dementia in approximately 15% of cases.

MND is characterised by degeneration of the motor nuclei in the cerebral cortex, brain stem and spinal cord, and of the corticobulbar and corticospinal tracts. Depending on the affected part of the motor system, MND is classified into amyotrophic lateral sclerosis (ALS), bulbar palsy, pseudobulbar palsy and progressive spinal muscular atrophy.

Clinical features
In all forms of MND, focal muscle weakness and painful muscle cramps are prominent features. Fasciculations are common. Some patients report sensory symptoms, such as tingling sensations and sensations of heat or cold. Depression and anxiety are common. The clinical features of MND can be either a mixture of upper and lower motor neuron signs (ALS), bulbar palsy, pseudobulbar palsy or a lower motor neuron syndrome (progressive spinal muscular atrophy). Approximately 50% of patients develop cognitive impairment. Dysphagia, weight loss and respiratory failure are common late complications.

The myelopathy of cervical spondylosis or cervical disc prolapse may be confused with ALS, and late-onset myopathies are sometimes difficult to distinguish from progressive muscle atrophy. The diagnosis of MND is confirmed with the presence of typical signs of muscle denervation on electromyography (see Chapter 2).

Treatment
Drug treatment of MND is not effective. To date, only Riluzole, a glutamate inhibitor, has been shown to influence the course of MND. It delays the need for mechanical ventilation and prolongs survival by approximately

3 months in patients who are less than 75 years old with good respiratory function (defined as a forced vital capacity more than 60%).

Although there is no curative treatment of MND at present, a well-coordinated management programme may alleviate suffering and improve the patient's quality of life. An important aim of such a programme is to prevent or delay the medical complications of MND and to manage them effectively when they arise. It should also maximise the patient's functional independence and provide practical and emotional support to patients and their carers. To this end, early counselling and advanced planning of care are essential. In particular, it is important to establish at the outset the patient's desire for life-sustaining interventions, such as gastrostomy tube feeding and ventilatory support. In the final stages of the disease, care is usually best provided by a palliative care team in the patient's own home or in a hospice.

Prognosis
MND is relentlessly progressive and the prognosis is generally poor. Disability occurs early and the average life expectancy is three years from the first symptoms. Longer survival occurs in young patients, when the respiratory function is relatively preserved, and in those with the ALS form of MND. The bulbar and pseudobulbar forms of MND have the worst prognosis.

CHAPTER 10

TUMOURS OF THE NERVOUS SYSTEM

Tumours of the nervous system account for only 2% of all primary tumours in adults. By contrast, one in five primary tumours in children occurs in the brain or the spinal cord. The causes of CNS tumours are not fully understood, but radiation to the neck and head and, in some families, genetic predisposition are known to increase the risk of brain tumours, including gliomas and meningiomas.

Most of the nervous system tumours occur in the brain. The spinal cord and the peripheral nervous system are affected less frequently. The most common primary brain tumours in adults are gliomas, primary CNS lymphomas, meningiomas, craniopharyngiomas, pituitary adenomas and ependymomas. Spread of metastases from other organs accounts for 9-17% of brain and spinal cord malignancy. Pilocytic astrocytomas, brain stem gliomas and embryonal tumours, e.g. medulloblastoma and craniopharyngiomas, are the most common neoplasms in children.

Clinical features of brain tumours

Patients with brain tumours may present with any combination of focal neurological signs, epileptic seizures, personality and behavioural changes, and cognitive impairment.

Diffuse infiltrative tumours that frequently affect the frontal and temporal lobes, such as gliomas and primary CNS lymphomas, initially result in cognitive impairment and changes in personality and behaviour, e.g. loss of emotional control, apathy, indifference or impulsiveness. Focal or generalised epileptic seizures, headaches, and anxiety and depression are also early features. Focal neurological signs are late manifestations of infiltrative brain tumours.

Presentation with focal neurological signs is also rare in the early stage of tumours that obstruct the CSF pathways, e.g. ependymoma of the fourth ventricle, craniopharyngioma and medulloblastoma. The early clinical presentation in these cases is usually with symptoms and signs of raised intracranial pressure.

Some tumours have a predilection for certain sites. For example, a tumour in the cerebellopontine angle is most likely to be either an acoustic neuroma, meningioma, an epidermoid cyst or a metastasis. Common tumours in the suprasellar region are pituitary adenomas, meningiomas and craniopharyngiomas. The initial clinical manifestation of these tumours is with focal neurological signs. The focal neurological signs depend on the site and size of the tumour and its growth rate.

The late clinical signs that are common to all brain tumours are those of raised intracranial pressure, displacement of adjacent structures, and temporal lobe-tentorial herniation or cerebellar-foramen magnum herniation. These complications occur when the tumour is large or has caused massive cerebral oedema or obstruction of the CSF pathways.

Diagnosis
As discussed in Chapter 1, analysis of the patient's symptoms and findings from the physical examination often suggest the site of the lesion. The tendency for certain tumours to occur in specific locations within the CNS and the differences in the clinical course of benign and malignant tumours are also useful in diagnosis.

It is often possible to distinguish between benign and malignant brain tumours from the clinical presentation. Benign tumours are usually slow growing, non-invasive or only locally invasive. They do not spread to other organs and do not cause systemic disease, such as weight loss, hypercalcaemia, paraneoplastic syndromes, etc. In all cases of suspected tumours, radiological and laboratory investigations are necessary.

Brain or spinal cord imaging is an essential part of the diagnostic workup of CNS tumours. CT and MRI scans with or without contrast enhancement are the first choice investigation in most cases. In addition to confirming the presence of a structural lesion and its site and size, imaging provides valuable information as to the nature of the tumour. For example, oedema surrounding the tumour and necrosis and/or haemorrhage within the tumour are an indication of the malignant nature of the tumour. On the other hand, a single mass lesion with clear borders suggests a benign tumour. The number of lesions also provides diagnostic clues. Multiple small lesions are more likely to be metastases than primary tumours.

Treatment decisions are based on establishing whether the tumour is benign or malignant, and, if malignant, its histological grade. Therefore, in addition to the findings of the history and clinical examination and imaging studies it is important to make a histological diagnosis. The tissue is usually obtained with a biopsy. In some cases, e.g. primary CNS lymphoma, malignant cells are sometimes found in the CSF.

Benign brain tumours

The most common benign brain tumours in adults are meningiomas, acoustic neuromas, pituitary adenomas and craniopharyngiomas.

Meningiomas

Meningiomas are the third most common brain tumours in adults. They originate from the arachnoidal cells of the leptomeninges. They are more common in females and their incidence increases with age. Traumatic brain injury, hormone replacement therapy, exposure to ionising radiation and old age are risk factors for developing meningiomas. The disease is sporadic, but there is also a rare familial form.

Meningiomas tend to occur in the suprasellar region, the olfactory groove of the anterior cranial fossa, the parasagittal area, the cerebellopontine angle, and the thoracic and cervical spinal cord. The clinical presentation depends on the location of the tumour.

Meningiomas are classified into benign (grade 1), atypical (grade 2) and anaplastic malignant (grade 3). Almost 90% of meningiomas are benign, slow-growing tumours. Malignant transformation of benign meningiomas is rare. Atypical and anaplastic meningiomas are locally invasive, aggressive tumours that often destroy the adjacent skull bones. They also tend to recur after treatment. Treatment of grade 1 meningiomas is surgical resection. In grades 2 and 3, radiotherapy is necessary in addition to total or subtotal surgical resection.

Pituitary adenomas
Pituitary adenomas arise from the adenohypophyseal cells. They account for 10-15% of all brain tumours. They are classified according to their size into microadenomas (diameter 10 mm or less) and macroadenomas. They are either hormone secreting or non-secreting. Three types of pituitary adenomas are distinguished on the basis of their morphological characteristics and clinical behaviour. These are benign adenomas, atypical adenomas and malignant adenomas (pituitary carcinomas). Most pituitary tumours are benign. Atypical adenomas are locally invasive and, like meningiomas, spread into the adjacent dura and bone. They frequently recur after surgical resection. Pituitary carcinomas are very rare.

The clinical features are due to pressure on local structures causing visual field defects (usually bitemporal hemianopia) or cranial nerve palsies, or due to the effects of excessive secretion of one or more pituitary hormones. Excessive secretion of prolactin, growth hormone, adrenocorticotrophic hormone (ACTH) and follicle-stimulating hormone (FSH) occurs in most patients.

Prolactin-secreting tumours (prolactinomas) are the most common type of pituitary adenomas. They cause secondary amenorrhoea and galactorrhoea; the severity of which is proportional to the size of the tumour. Growth-hormone-secreting tumours result in acromegaly (or gigantism if they occur before puberty), and tumours that secrete ACTH result in Cushing's disease (truncal obesity, hypertension, proximal muscle weakness, hirsutism and osteoporosis).

Surgical resection of the tumour is sufficient in cases of benign adenomas except prolactin-secreting adenomas, which usually respond to treatment with dopamine agonists, such as cabergoline. Treatment of atypical adenomas and pituitary carcinomas consists of a combination of surgical excision and radiotherapy.

Craniopharyngiomas

Craniopharyngiomas are embryonal, slow-growing tumours. The tumour is solid, cystic, partially calcified and occurs in the sella turcica or parasellar region. It has a bimodal age distribution. Half the cases are diagnosed in childhood or adolescence. In adults the peak age of presentation is 50 to 75 years.

The tumour usually invades the pituitary gland and hypothalamus, and causes pressure on the optic chiasma or optic nerve. Children present with headaches, weight gain, diabetes insipidus, low growth rate, delayed puberty and visual field defects. The appearance of the MRI scans is typical and demonstrates the presence of a solid, cystic and partially calcified tumour in the region of the sella turcica. Endocrine tests provide evidence of hormonal deficiencies.

Treatment is total tumour resection if there is no involvement of the hypothalamus and the visual pathways. In cases where the latter structures are affected, the treatment of choice is limited surgical resection that spares the hypothalamus and optic chiasma and subsequent radiotherapy.

The prognosis for survival is good. Approximately 70% of patients survive 20 years or more after treatment. However, the tumour recurrence rate after surgery is high and endocrine dysfunction is common.

Craniopharyngiomas in adults cause panhypopituitarism, visual disturbances, mental confusion and, in some cases, signs of raised intracranial pressure.

Acoustic neuromas

Acoustic neuromas (also called vestibular schwannomas) are benign tumours that arise from Schwann cells of the myelin sheath of the vestibular division of the vestibulocochlear (VIII) nerve. Very rarely the tumour arises from the cochlear division. They account for 90% of all tumours in the cerebellopontine angle. The peak incidence of acoustic neuromas is the fifth decade of life. The cause of the tumour is unknown. There has been speculation that the frequent use of mobile telephones might increase the risk of developing acoustic neuromas, but there is no evidence of this at present.

Acoustic neuromas are almost always unilateral. Bilateral acoustic neuromas occur rarely in patients with neurofibromatosis. The earliest symptoms are unilateral tinnitus and gradual asymmetrical sensorineural hearing loss. As the tumour size increases, the symptoms and signs usually evolve in the following sequence: vertigo and ataxia, facial pain, V, VII and IX cranial nerve palsies, raised intracranial pressure, and epileptic seizures.

The treatment of first choice is surgery. Radiotherapy is an option when surgery is contraindicated.

Malignant brain tumours

Approximately 60 to 80% of all malignant brain tumours are gliomas. The second most common malignant brain tumour is primary non-Hodgkin's CNS lymphoma.

GLIOMAS

Gliomas are common CNS malignancies. They arise from glial cells, i.e. astrocytes, oligodendrocytes and ependymal cells. Gliomas are most frequently diagnosed in middle age. They tend to occur in the frontal and temporal lobes, the cerebellum, and the brain stem. Two subtypes of gliomas, namely astrocytomas and ependymomas, also occur in the spinal cord and are usually intramedullary. Classification of gliomas is clinically useful for the choice of treatment. It also provides prognostic information.

Gliomas are classified according to their histological characteristics and degree of malignancy into four grades (WHO classification, 2007). Grade I astrocytoma is a solid, non-infiltrative, well-differentiated, low-grade tumour. It has the best prognosis, although 70% of cases are transformed into a high-grade tumour within 5-10 years. Treatment is subtotal surgical resection. The 5-year survival rate is 50%.

Grades II (oligodendroglioma), III (anaplastic oligoastrocytoma) and IV (glioblastoma) are diffuse infiltrating gliomas. In contrast to grade I tumours (astrocytomas), they infiltrate the brain tissue and have no clear demarcation from the surrounding healthy structures. More than 80% of gliomas are of this type. The high-grade diffuse infiltrating gliomas (grade III and IV) carry a poor prognosis. Treatment is by a combination of total or maximal surgical resection, radiotherapy and chemotherapy. Less than 5% of patients survive 5 years after the diagnosis.

A particularly aggressive form of glioma known as diffuse intrinsic pontine glioma occurs in children. The mean age of diagnosis is 7 years. Treatment is with radiotherapy, but is usually ineffective. Most patients die within a year of diagnosis.

PRIMARY CNS LYMPHOMAS (PCNSL)

PCNSL are non-Hodgkin's B-cell diffuse, infiltrative malignant tumours. The disease affects the brain, spinal cord, eyes, cranial nerves and meninges. PCNSL are rare compared to gliomas except in immunocompromised patients, e.g. those with AIDS/HIV or organ transplants. Only 3-5% of all brain tumours are PCNSL. The incidence in immunocompetent patients increases with age.

The clinical presentation is similar to that of gliomas. The diagnosis is made in most cases with MRI scans and stereotactic biopsy. In some patients the malignant cells are present in the CSF. Treatment is with a combination of chemotherapy and whole brain radiotherapy. Old age, immunodeficiency and early relapses are poor prognostic factors.

Metastatic brain tumours

Secondary spread of cancer to the brain is common. It has been estimated that between 20% and 40% of patients with cancer develop brain metastases. This high incidence is probably due to the improved survival of cancer patients. The most common tumours that metastasise to the brain are breast carcinoma, melanoma and carcinoma of the lung.

One in four cases of metastatic brain tumours is due to breast carcinoma. The metastases are usually multiple, and frequently spread to the frontal lobes and cerebellum. The most common symptoms are headaches, vomiting, visual disturbances and epileptic seizures.

Approximately 50% of patients with melanomas develop brain metastases. The metastases are usually multiple and are associated with poor prognosis. The average survival after metastatic spread to the brain is one year.

More than a third of brain metastases are due to carcinoma of the lung. In half the cases there is just one metastatic tumour. Treatment of solitary metastases is with stereotactic neurosurgery. Solitary lesions have a better prognosis than multiple metastases and, with treatment, the survival is usually more than a year. The treatment of multiple metastases is whole brain radiotherapy; the mean survival time is 4-6 months.

Carcinoma of the prostate and multiple myeloma metastasise to the skull bones. These tumours are often asymptomatic for long periods except when they involve the base of the skull and cause cranial nerve palsies. Other tumours that spread to the brain include osteosarcoma and colorectal carcinoma.

The treatment modalities for brain metastases are whole brain radiotherapy, stereotactic radiotherapy and surgery. The choice of a treatment method depends on the number and site of the metastatic tumours, the general health of the patient and status of the primary tumour. For example, surgery or stereotactic radiotherapy is usually the treatment of choice for a single metastasis, especially if it is in the posterior fossa and likely to cause obstruction of the CSF pathways and hydrocephalus. Whole brain radiotherapy is used for the treatment of multiple metastases. The prognosis of brain metastases is generally poor.

Tumours of the spinal cord

Tumours of the spinal cord are rare compared to brain tumours. They account for less than a fifth of all tumours of the nervous system. Their location is either intramedullary or extramedullary. The extramedullary tumour are either extradural or intradural.

Most spinal cord tumours are extradural extramedullary. They arise from the vertebrae and epidural tissues, or are metastases. The most common extradural tumours are metastatic lymphomas, myelomas and bronchogenic carcinoma.

The second most common group of spinal cord tumours are extramedullary and intradural. Their origin is the leptomeninges and the nerve roots. Neurofibromas and meningiomas constitute the majority of these tumours.

The clinical manifestations of the extramedullary tumours is that of slowly progressive spinal cord compression resulting in asymmetrical spastic paraparesis or tetraparesis with a sensory level and bladder and bowel dysfunction, or a cauda equina or conus medullaris syndrome. Involvement of the nerve roots results in a painful radiculopathy with typical segmental sensory and motor features. The differential diagnosis of extramedullary tumours includes cervical spondylosis (with myelopathy), spinal abscess, tuberculous granulomas and a prolapsed intervertebral disc.

Tumours within the spinal cord itself, i.e. intramedullary, are rare and are mostly ependymomas or astrocytomas. They give rise to symptoms and signs of syringomyelia.

The diagnosis of spinal tumours consists of confirming the site and extent of the tumour and its histopathological type and grade. MRI scans are the preferred imaging technique for determining the location and size of the tumour. The histopathological diagnosis is usually made during surgery to enable the selection of the appropriate surgical procedure. Total resection of the visible tumour is the optimal treatment in cases of low-grade malignancy. Radiotherapy and/or chemotherapy are/is usually the treatment for high-grade malignancy.

Tumours of the peripheral nerves

The most common peripheral nerve tumours are schwannomas, neurofibromas, and neurogenic sarcomas (also called malignant peripheral nerve tumours). A peripheral nerve tumour should be distinguished from a ganglion or an intraneural lipoma. Ganglions are mucin and synovial fluid-filled small cysts that occur near a joint or ligament. Their most common site is the dorsum of the hand.

Schwannomas are benign tumours that arise from Schwann cells of the myelin sheath. In 25% of cases schwannomas occur in the head and neck region. The peak age of onset is 30-40 years.

Neurofibromas are also benign tumours that are predominantly made of perineural cells but also contain fibroblasts and Schwann cells. Neurofibromas can be either solitary or multiple tumours. The latter are usually one of the manifestations of neurofibromatosis (von Recklinghausen disease). Neurofibromas usually occur in the skin. Non-cutaneous neurofibromas are rare. The tumour is solid, well-defined and slow growing. The clinical signs depend on the site of the neurofibroma and are mainly due to compression of adjacent structures. The diagnosis is confirmed with biopsy. Treatment of symptomatic peripheral nerve tumours is surgical resection. Tumour recurrence is very rare.

Paraneoplastic neurological disorders

Malignant tumours of the lungs, breast, ovaries and other organs may cause immune-mediated, non-metastatic syndromes that can affect either the central or peripheral nervous system. These are collectively known as the paraneoplastic neurological disorders. They include immune disorders of the neuromuscular junction (e.g. Eaton-Lambert syndrome), polymyositis, dermatomyositis, peripheral neuropathies, limbic encephalitis, cerebellar degeneration, and others. Paraneoplastic syndromes may develop before or after the first clinical manifestations of the primary tumour. Recognition of these disorders is important because most respond well to treatment with intravenous immunoglobulins, corticosteroids or plasma exchange.

CHAPTER 11

DISEASES OF THE PERIPHERAL NERVOUS SYSTEM

The main disorders of the peripheral nervous system (PNS) are neuropathies, radiculopathies, trauma and tumours. (PNS tumours and trauma are described in Chapters 10 and 14, respectively.)

Peripheral neuropathies

The term peripheral neuropathy is used to describe damage to a peripheral nerve or nerves irrespective of the underlying cause. Clinical entities that result from disorders of the anterior horn cells (e.g. poliomyelitis) or the sensory ganglia (e.g. herpes zoster) are called motor or sensory neuronopathies respectively, and are not included in the definition of a peripheral neuropathy.

Peripheral neuropathies can be focal or generalised. In focal neuropathies the pathological process may affect a single nerve (mononeuropathy), or more than one nerve in different parts of the body either simultaneously or sequentially, i.e. multiple mononeuropathy (also called mononeuritis multiplex). In generalised, i.e. polyneuropathy, the pathological process in the peripheral nerves is symmetrical, usually affects the lower limbs more than the upper limbs, and starts in the distal part of the limb and, as the disease worsens, progresses proximally.

The pathological changes of a peripheral neuropathy can predominantly affect either the axon (axonal degeneration), the myelin sheath (demyelination), or both. The autonomic nervous system may also be affected. In contrast to neuropathies, trauma resulting in transection of a healthy peripheral nerve causes Wallerian degeneration: a process in which both the axon and the myelin sheath degenerate distal to the site of transection with subsequent slow, and usually incomplete, recovery. (Wallerian degeneration is also rarely caused by acute ischaemic nerve injury.)

The extent of the pathological changes in the myelin sheath or the axon has important prognostic significance. In demyelinating (sensory) neuropathies the recovery, i.e. remyelination, is often complete and usually occurs in days or weeks. The opposite is true for most axonal (motor) neuropathies. Patients with sensory or motor polyneuropathy may also have symptoms of autonomic system dysfunction.

Aetiology

The most common causes of peripheral neuropathy are diabetes mellitus (see Chapter 13), chronic excessive alcohol consumption, Guillain-Barré syndrome, and non-metastatic paraneoplastic syndromes associated with malignant tumours. (Leprosy is the leading cause of neuropathy in some countries.) Other important, but less frequent, causes are systemic vasculitis (e.g. due to connective tissue disease, such as systemic lupus erythematosus or rheumatoid arthritis), AIDS, vitamin B12 deficiency (the neuropathy often coexists with subacute combined degeneration of the spinal cord), uraemia, drug toxicity (e.g. pyridoxine, metronidazole, nitrofurantoin, ethambutol, isoniazid, amiodarone, phenytoin) and hereditary polyneuropathies. A common cause of mononeuropathies is compression or entrapment by tumours or local anatomical structures.

Clinical features of polyneuropathy

The onset of polyneuropathy is either acute, subacute or chronic. Dysaesthesia is usually the first symptom. Typically, the patient complains of tingling, 'pins and needles' or numbness in the toes of both feet and the tips of fingers. Reduced manual dexterity and a tendency to trip over when walking are also early features. The legs are usually affected before the hands and, as a rule, more severely. At this stage the clinical examination may reveal loss of the ankle jerk, weakness of dorsiflexion of the toes and mild symmetrical impairment of all sensory modalities.

As the disease progresses, the dysaesthesia and the impairment of skin sensation spread more proximally in the upper and lower limbs: a pattern often described as 'glove and stocking distribution'. Examination confirms bilateral foot drop and loss of the ankle and knee jerks. In severe polyneuropathy, sensory ataxia and muscle atrophy are also present and cause significant functional disability. Neuropathic pain is a prominent feature of some polyneuropathies.

Autonomic neuropathy

Autonomic neuropathy occurs without symptoms and signs of sensory or motor neuropathy in some rare genetically-determined disorders. However, more frequently, it coexists with polyneuropathy (e.g. in alcoholics and in patients with chronic renal failure), Guillain-Barré syndrome, paraneoplastic syndromes and diabetes mellitus. The main features of autonomic neuropathy are postural hypotension, supine hypertension, bradycardia, anhidrosis, erectile dysfunction, diarrhoea or constipation.

Mononeuropathy and multiple mononeuropathy

Damage of a single nerve (mononeuropathy) is most frequently due to nerve compression, e.g. in the carpal tunnel. Diabetes mellitus, vasculitis associated with connective tissue disease (such as systemic lupus erythematosus), malignancy and AIDS/HIV infection are the most common causes of multiple mononeuropathy.

Diagnosis

Nerve conduction studies and electromyography are the main tests used to confirm the diagnosis of peripheral neuropathy and to distinguish axonal from demyelinating neuropathy. In axonal neuropathy, the motor unit action potentials are reduced but the nerve conduction velocity is either normal or slightly reduced. Demyelination, on the other hand, causes significant reduction in the conduction velocity, usually to 40% or less of the normal value.

Nerve biopsy is rarely needed to establish the aetiology of the neuropathy. It is indicated in cases of undiagnosed severe chronic progressive polyneuropathy.

Differential diagnosis

The first step in the differential diagnosis is to exclude spinal cord lesions and radiculopathies that mimic polyneuropathy. Once the diagnosis of polyneuropathy is confirmed, its cause should be ascertained.

Diseases of the spinal cord are sometimes difficult to distinguish from polyneuropathies. However, the typical symmetrical distribution of the clinical signs in polyneuropathy is often helpful in the differential diagnosis. As a rule, asymmetrical symptoms and signs suggest a diagnosis other than a polyneuropathy, such as cauda equina lesions or myelitis. In these cases, electrophysiological studies and radiological tests are often required to rule out these disorders.

The causes of peripheral neuropathies are numerous but can be narrowed down to only a few by the careful evaluation of the history and clinical findings. For example, a neuropathy that is progressive over a number of years is often a hereditary or diabetic neuropathy. In such cases, the medical and family history and the presence of other signs, e.g. claw toes or pes cavus, further supports the diagnosis of a hereditary neuropathy. Similarly, the presence of symptoms and signs of systemic disease provides valuable diagnostic clues. Laboratory investigations are an important part of the diagnostic workup of neuropathies. The minimum screening tests should include measurement of the fasting blood glucose, vitamin B12, a full blood count and serum protein electrophoresis.

Treatment

Treatment of the underlying cause and the control of pain and other symptoms are the mainstay of the management of peripheral neuropathies.

Guillain-Barré syndrome (GBS)

GBS (also known as acute demyelinating polyradiculoneuropathy) is an immune-mediated acute or subacute sensorimotor inflammatory disorder of the peripheral nervous system (PNS). There is also a chronic relapsing form of the disease and a variant known as Miller Fisher syndrome. GBS is characterised by acute extensive inflammatory changes of the PNS. The anterior nerve roots are more severely affected. The main pathological changes are demyelination and axonal degeneration.

Clinical features

GBS is frequently preceded by an acute infection, usually an upper respiratory tract infection. The onset is acute or subacute with distal dysesthesias and distal muscle weakness. The muscle weakness spreads quickly (usually in 2 or 3 days). It affects the proximal muscles of the upper and lower limbs. Less frequently, the weakness starts in the neck and shoulder muscles and spreads distally. The tendon reflexes are absent and there is mild impairment of skin sensation. Facial nerve palsy and dysphagia occur in more than 50% of cases. Mild or moderately severe neuropathic pain is also common. The patient usually develops significant functional disability within 2-4 weeks of the disease onset. Respiratory muscle weakness and symptoms of autonomic system dysfunction are common in severe cases and affect one in every three patients with GBS. In the Miller Fisher variant of GBS there is also ataxia, and ophthalmoplegia.

The differential diagnosis of GBS includes myelopathy, cauda equina syndrome, muscle disease and botulism.

Diagnosis

Nerve conduction studies demonstrate evidence of a motor and sensory neuropathy with small motor unit action potentials and slow nerve conduction velocity that is more severe in the spinal nerve roots segment. CSF protein is raised and the CSF cell content is usually normal.

Management

Careful monitoring of the respiratory and autonomic system function, prevention of deep vein thrombosis, and supportive care are essential in all cases of GBS. Severe hypoxia is an indication for intubation and artificial ventilation. Hypotension, cardiac arrhythmias and other symptoms of autonomic dysfunction require prompt treatment.

Intravenous immunoglobulins or plasma exchange are the treatments of first choice in severe GBS and should usually be given in the first two weeks. Corticosteroids are not effective except when combined with immunoglobulins.

Prognosis

The prognosis of GBS is generally good. Approximately 80% of patients show complete or almost complete recovery in 6 months or less. The disease is usually monophasic and recurrence is rare. Approximately 10-15% of survivors continue to have a significant long-term disability.

The mortality rate of GBS is low. A rapid onset and severe muscle weakness within a few hours, old age and the need for respiratory support are poor prognostic factors.

Chronic inflammatory demyelinating polyradiculoneuropathy

This is a chronic relapsing or slowly progressive sensorimotor neuropathy. In contrast to classical GBS, respiratory failure and involvement of the autonomic nervous system are rare. Treatment is with corticosteroids and the prognosis is good in most cases.

Entrapment neuropathies

Entrapment neuropathies result from compression and/or traction of peripheral nerves that pass through narrow anatomical structures. The most common entrapment neuropathies are the carpal tunnel and cubital tunnel syndromes.

Carpal tunnel syndrome

The carpal tunnel is the narrow groove between the wrist bones on the palmar side of the hand. It is covered by the retinaculum flexorum. The median nerve and several tendons pass through the carpal tunnel. Compression of the median nerve in this area results in the carpal tunnel syndrome (CTS).

The causes of the CTS include diabetes mellitus, arthritis, hypothyroidism, obesity and occupational injury (e.g. the frequent use of vibrating tools or tasks that require repetitive wrist flexion).

The median nerve innervates the muscles of the thenar eminence and the skin of the thumb, index, middle finger and the lateral half of the ring finger. However, minor anatomical variations between individuals are common. The clinical features of CTS are a combination of pain, skin sensory changes and muscle weakness.

The earliest symptoms are dysaesthesia and pain typically affecting the thumb, index and middle fingers, and the lateral half of the ring finger. However, some patients report pain in all fingers and also in the forearm. The symptoms are usually more severe at night. The pain is frequently described as 'like an electric shock'. Occasionally, the sensory symptoms and signs are very mild or completely absent. In severe cases the patient develops wasting and weakness of the thenar muscles and skin sensory loss in the above-described distribution. Tinel's sign is often positive. (Tinel's sign is positive when pressure on the retinaculum flexorum or tapping over it causes tingling and pins and needles in the skin area innervated by the median nerve.) The diagnosis of CTS is confirmed with electromyography and nerve conduction studies.

The initial treatment of CTS is with splinting at night and local steroid injections. In severe cases, or when conservative treatment is unsuccessful, surgical decompression is indicated.

Cubital tunnel syndrome

The cubital tunnel is the narrow gap between the medial epicondyle and the olecranon that is covered by the cubital tunnel retinaculum and contains the ulnar nerve. Compression of the ulnar nerve in the cubital tunnel is usually caused by trauma due to repetitive elbow flexion. The cubital tunnel syndrome may also occur in patients with diabetes mellitus.

The ulnar nerve innervates the lumbrical muscles and the skin of the small finger and the medial aspect of the ring finger. Compression of the ulnar nerve in the cubital tunnel causes tingling, pins and needles, skin sensory loss in the small and ring fingers, and weakness and wasting of all small muscles of the hand, except the abductor pollicis brevis. Clawing of the small and ring fingers occurs in severe cases. In some patients there is also thickening and tenderness of the ulnar nerve at the elbow.

As with CTS, the diagnosis is confirmed with electrophysiological tests, and the treatment is conservative (splinting and local steroid injections) or surgical.

Radiculopathies

The radiculopathies are painful disorders of the spinal nerve roots. They are usually due to degenerative disease of the cervical and lumbar spine. Old age and spinal canal stenosis (defined as an anteroposterior spinal canal diameter less 10 mm) are the main predisposing factors. The pathological changes consist of a combination of facet joint hypertrophy, thickening of the spinal ligaments, osteophyte formation, degeneration of the intervertebral discs, and spondylolisthesis. These changes may result in the compression of the cervical or lumbar nerve roots, or the cauda equina.

Cervical radiculopathy

Cervical radiculopathy is characterised by neck and shoulder pain that radiates to one or both arms in a dermatome distribution and is due to nerve root irritation or compression. The disease is very common and its incidence and prevalence rise with increasing age. The most frequently affected nerve roots are C5, C6 and C7. Cervical radiculopathy is caused by degenerative arthritis (cervical spondylosis) in 75% of all cases. Acute cervical disc prolapse accounts for most of the remaining cases.

Acute disc prolapse occurs either in a patient with pre-existing cervical spondylosis following a neck flexion-extension injury, or following sports injury in a person without degenerative disease of the spine. Cervical spondylolisthesis (the forward displacement of a vertebra relative to the adjacent vertebrae and associated disc degeneration and facet joint hypertrophic arthropathy) is a rare cause of cervical radiculopathy and usually affects C3-C4 or C4-C5. Spondylolisthesis is more common in the lumbar region.

Clinical features

In addition to pain in the typical root sensory dermatome, the patient often complains of pins and needles in the upper limb. Neck pain is also common. Impairment or loss of skin sensation in one or more dermatomes may be present. However, the dermatomal distribution of the sensory symptoms and signs is not always helpful for the identification of the level of the lesion because of the overlap of the peripheral nerve territories of the upper limb.

Muscle weakness and wasting in a myotome distribution and depressed tendon reflexes are present in severe cases. Lesions of C5 cause weakness of the deltoid, supraspinatus and infraspinatus leading to weakness of shoulder abduction and external rotation, and loss of the biceps jerk. Lesions of C6 result in weakness of the biceps and brachioradialis muscles, weak elbow flexion and wrist flexion and extension, and absent supinator jerk.

Neck movements are painful and restricted. Spurling's test is often positive. (Spurling's test consists of turning the patient's head to the affected side and pressing on it. The test is positive if this manoeuvre reproduces the neuropathic pain and paraesthesia.)

Diagnosis
X-rays of the cervical spine demonstrate degenerative changes. However, because such changes are very common in older people they should be interpreted in conjunction with the clinical symptoms and signs. In cases of spondylolisthesis, a neck flexion-extension X-ray confirms the forward displacement of the affected vertebra. MRI scans are the imaging method of choice. EMG and nerve conduction studies are helpful in excluding other pathology.

Treatment
Conservative treatment with analgesics, rest and neck immobilisation with a cervical collar is effective in approximately 90% of patients. Surgical decompression is usually indicated if the symptoms persist after 6-8 weeks of conservative treatment and if there is a progressive neurological deficit.

Cervical spondylosis
Cervical spondylosis is a common disorder in middle-aged and elderly people. It results from degenerative changes in the intervertebral discs and ligaments. Congenital or acquired spinal canal stenosis is sometimes

present, especially in patients presenting with myelopathy. In most cases the disease affects multiple discs, usually C5 and C6.

Cervical spondylosis may result in a radiculopathy, a slowly progressive myelopathy, or myeloradiculopathy. The clinical features are variable and depend on the extent and severity of the disease. In advanced cases, patients present with spastic paraparesis and lower motor neuron weakness and wasting of the hand muscles. Neck extension often causes electric shock-like sensations and paraesthesia is the upper limbs (Lhermitte's sign).

The differential diagnosis includes motor neurone disease, spinal cord tumours and multiple sclerosis. The diagnosis is confirmed with cervical MRI scans and electromyography. Conservative treatment with analgesics and neck immobilisation (with a cervical collar) is effective in 75% of cases. A progressive neurological deficit or poor response to medical treatment is indication for surgery.

Lumbar radiculopathy

Chronic low back pain is one of the most common causes of disability and absence from work. Its main causes are lumbar disc degenerative disease without disc herniation or facet joint pathology (discogenic pain), congenital or acquired lumbar canal stenosis, disc prolapse and spondylolisthesis. The clinical manifestation of these pathological processes are radiculopathy and neurogenic claudication. Rarely, patients present with a cauda equina syndrome.

Degenerative disc disease of the lumbar spine usually causes radiculopathy of L5 and S1 roots. It is very rare for other lumbar nerve roots to be affected. Both L5 and S1 cause neuropathic pain in the back of the thigh, which radiates into the lateral aspect of the leg into the foot. The only distinguishing feature is that the pain involves the dorsal and ventral aspects of the foot in L5 radiculopathy, whereas the pain and sensory symptoms due to S1 lesions are confined to the lateral part of the foot. Muscle weakness and sensory signs are usually absent. The ankle jerk is depressed or absent in S1 disc prolapse.

Neurogenic claudication is characterised by radicular leg pain, numbness and leg weakness on standing and walking. These symptoms usually occur in a patient with long-standing low back pain. The distance that the patient can walk before the onset of pain becomes progressively shorter as the severity of the disease increases. The pain is usually bilateral and is relieved by rest, sitting and leaning forward. In contrast to vascular claudication, the pain is not in the calf. It has a dermatome distribution that corresponds to one or more nerve roots.

The diagnosis is based on the history and clinical examination and is confirmed with radiological investigations (plain X-ray films, CT or MRI scans). Neurophysiological studies are useful when an alternative diagnosis, e.g. lumbar plexopathy, cannot be excluded.

The initial treatment of choice of lumbar radiculopathy is conservative with analgesics, anticonvulsants and antidepressants, and physiotherapy. Fluoroscopically directed epidural injections are usually effective in severe cases. Failure of conservative treatment and a progressive neurological deficit are indications for surgical decompression.

CHAPTER 12

MUSCLE DISORDERS

Muscle diseases can be grouped into five categories. These are idiopathic inflammatory myopathies, hereditary myopathies, metabolic and endocrine myopathies, myopathies due to alcohol misuse and drug toxicity, and diseases of the neuromuscular junction. Although muscle weakness is a characteristic feature of all myopathies, these disorders differ from each other in many respects. The main differentiating features are the patient's age at the time of the disease onset, the distribution of muscle weakness, the course of the disease, the presence or absence of systemic symptoms, and the histopathological findings on muscle biopsy.

Idiopathic inflammatory myopathies

The idiopathic inflammatory myopathies are immune-mediated disorders of unknown cause. They are polymyositis, dermatomyositis, inclusion body myositis, and necrotising myopathy. Necrotising myopathy is very rare and is not discussed further in this book. The incidence of the idiopathic inflammatory myopathies is 4-5 new cases per 100,000 of the population per year. Polymyositis is the most common of these disorders.

Polymyositis

Polymyositis is a symmetrical painless inflammatory proximal myopathy that predominantly affects older people. Its peak incidence is in those 50 to 60 years old. It is more common in females. In older people, the disease may be associated with malignancy, especially carcinoma of the lung, colon, breast and ovary.

The disease onset may be acute or insidious. The patient presents with symptoms suggestive of weakness of the proximal limb muscles, e.g.

inability to rise from a low chair or to raise the arms above the shoulder. The muscle weakness is usually slowly progressive. Muscle pain (myalgia) is rare, and muscle wasting is a late feature and is usually mild or moderately severe. The extra ocular muscles are never affected. Systemic symptoms, including low-grade fever, anorexia and weight loss, are common. The erythrocyte sedimentation rate (ESR) and the C-reactive protein (CRP) are raised.

Dermatomyositis

The clinical features of dermatomyositis are similar to those of polymyositis but, in addition, there are typical skin lesions. A malignant tumour is present in a third of patients with late-onset dermatomyositis.

The skin involvement may occur any time during the course of the disease. Frequently, there is a localised or diffuse macular rash. In typical cases the skin rash is found on the bridge of the nose and forehead, and on the knuckles, elbows and knees. In some cases V-shaped erythematous rash on the neck is present. An eczema-like rash or extensive exfoliative dermatitis may also occur.

Inclusion body myositis

Approximately 25% of all cases of the idiopathic inflammatory myopathies are due to inclusion body myositis. It is the most common inflammatory myopathy in older people.

Inclusion body myositis is characterised by painless, slowly progressive, usually asymmetrical weakness of the proximal and distal muscles. Dysphagia occurs in more than 50% of patients. Muscle cramps are rare.

Treatment of polymyositis and dermatomyositis is with corticosteroids alone, or in combination with either azathioprine or methotrexate. When this drug combination is not effective, intravenous immunoglobulins are an alternative second-line treatment. There is no effective treatment at present for inclusion body myositis.

The prognosis of the idiopathic inflammatory myopathies is generally good. Long remissions occur in most cases except when the disease is associated with malignant tumours.

The congenital and hereditary myopathies

The congenital myopathies are characterised by a genetically-determined failure of muscle development, and include a large group of progressive and non-progressive disorders. The main symptom of the congenital myopathies is hypotonia, which is present from birth or early infancy. (This is frequently referred to as the floppy infant syndrome.) Skeletal abnormalities, e.g. pes cavus or scoliosis, are common.

The most common hereditary myopathies of childhood are Duchenne and Becker's muscular dystrophies. Myotonic dystrophy is the most common myopathy in adults.

Duchenne and Becker's muscular dystrophies

Duchenne muscular dystrophy is a sex-linked muscle disease that results from mutation of the dystrophin gene and has a prevalence of 3 cases per 100,000. (Dystrophin is a cytoplasmic muscle protein that, in conjunction with other proteins, strengthens the muscle fibre and maintains its anatomical integrity.) The disease affects boys and its onset is in early childhood. (Girls with Turner's syndrome, i.e. XO genotype, may also be affected.)

The first manifestation of the disease is usually between the ages of 3 and 6 years. The proximal pelvic girdle muscles are affected first. The child develops difficulties ascending stairs, rising from the floor and walking. A characteristic feature of the disease is hypertrophy of the calf muscles. The muscle weakness and wasting is relatively rapidly progressive. Some degree of learning disability is usually present.

The prognosis of Duchenne muscular dystrophy is poor. By the age of 12 years, most children are unable to walk and are severely disabled. Life expectancy is 20-30 years. Death is usually due to infections, or respiratory or heart failure.

Becker's muscular dystrophy is clinically similar to Duchenne's, but the disease is more benign. It is also sex-linked but, in contrast to Duchenne's muscular dystrophy, dystrophin is not completely absent. The onset is in late childhood and the disability due to the weakness usually occurs in the third decade of life. Most patients live beyond middle age.

Myotonic dystrophy

Myotonic dystrophy is the most common hereditary myopathy in adult life. It has a prevalence of 1:8,000. The mode of inheritance is autosomal dominant with high penetrance. The muscle weakness may be present at birth (congenital form), or starts in childhood, early or late adult life. In most cases the symptoms start in the third decade of life. Three clinical features distinguish myotonic dystrophy from other myopathies: the distribution of the muscle weakness, the presence of myotonia, and the presence of pathology in organs other than the musculoskeletal system.

The muscle weakness and wasting is progressive and affects the distal limb muscles, and the neck and facial muscles. The masseters, temporalis and levator palpebrae superioris muscles are always affected resulting in the typical hatchet facial appearance and bilateral ptosis. The sternomastoid and forearm muscles are also affected early in the course of myotonic dystrophy. Dysphagia and respiratory muscle weakness occur in the later stages of the disease.

Myotonia is characterised by the delayed relaxation of muscles after a strong voluntary contraction. For example, the patient may have difficulty releasing his grip on objects. The myotonia may precede or follow the muscle weakness. It is usually aggravated by cold, exercise and fasting.

In addition to the muscle weakness and myotonia, patients with myotonic dystrophy often have cardiac conduction defects, cataracts, hypogonadism (gynaecomastia and testicular atrophy), diabetes mellitus and cognitive deficits.

The course of myotonic dystrophy is slowly progressive. Life expectancy is normal or slightly reduced.

The metabolic and endocrine myopathies

The metabolic myopathies result from disorders of the utilisation of carbohydrates and fat in muscle and other organs. This group of myopathies is rare and is caused by the glycogen storage diseases and lipid storage diseases. These diseases result from defects in the genes that code for various enzymes involved in carbohydrate and lipid metabolism, and the symptoms are present from early childhood.

Diseases of the endocrine system can also result in myopathies. Patients with severe thyrotoxicosis may develop a chronic proximal myopathy, extra ocular muscle weakness (exophthalmic ophthalmoplegia) and, rarely, episodic muscle paralysis that usually lasts several hours and resolves spontaneously. Proximal myopathy also occurs in Cushing's disease and acromegaly.

Myopathies due to alcohol and drug toxicity

Alcohol-induced myopathy

Two types of alcohol-induced myopathy may be distinguished: acute and chronic. Acute alcoholic myopathy usually follows a bout of binge drinking and results in rhabdomyolysis. There is severe muscle pain. Muscle tenderness and weakness are also prominent features. Laboratory investigations confirm the presence of severe hypokalaemia, myoglobinuria, raised serum creatinine phosphokinase (CPK), and evidence of impaired renal function or overt acute renal failure. Severe cases are life-threatening. However, partial recovery usually occurs with treatment and abstinence from alcohol.

Chronic alcoholic myopathy is characterised by a painless, predominantly proximal muscle weakness. Muscle cramps are common. Hypokalaemia may be present and the serum CPK is either raised or normal. Chronic alcoholic myopathy may be initially asymptomatic. However, the disease is slowly progressive, and three out of every four patients develop a clinically significant myopathy after years of heavy sustained alcohol misuse. This type of myopathy responds less well to treatment (correction of potassium deficiency, rehydration and supportive medical care) and permanent residual disability is common.

Myopathy due to prescription drugs

Statins and the fibrate lipid lowering drugs, and corticosteroids may cause a painful, usually proximal weakness and muscle tenderness. The CPK is usually elevated, but is sometimes within the normal limits. The onset may be acute or insidious, and the occurrence of the myopathy has no relation to the duration of treatment or the dose.

Several drugs block the acetylcholine neurotransmission at the neuromuscular junction resulting in episodic muscle weakness. This group of drugs includes penicillamine, the aminoglycoside antibiotics (e.g. streptomycin, gentamycin, etc.), and the anti-malarial drugs chloroquine, quinine and quinidine.

Disorders of the neuromuscular junction

This group of muscle disease is characterised by episodic and recurrent failure of neurotransmission at the neuromuscular junction that causes temporary muscle weakness. The most important disorder in this group is myasthenia gravis. A rare non-metastatic paraneoplastic syndrome, usually associated with oat cell carcinoma of the lung and known as Eaton-Lambert syndrome, and severe hereditary or acquired hypokalaemia also cause episodic skeletal muscle weakness.

Myasthenia gravis

Myasthenia gravis is a rare autoimmune disease. Its incidence and prevalence respectively are 10-20 and 200 cases per million. The onset is usually in the second or third decade of life. In some cases the onset is after the age of 60 years. There is also a congenital form of myasthenia gravis. The disease is more common in females. It results from the immune destruction of the acetylcholine receptors in the postsynaptic membrane of the neuromuscular junction. The thymus gland has an important role in the pathogenesis of myasthenia gravis, and approximately 10% of patients have a thymoma. Most of the remaining patients have thymus hyperplasia. There is also a high incidence of thyrotoxicosis, hypothyroidism, diabetes mellitus, vitiligo and connective tissue diseases in patients with myasthenia gravis.

A triad of features distinguish myasthenia gravis from other muscle diseases:

1. The muscle weakness is episodic and occurs as a result of continued muscle activity.
2. The muscle strength is quickly restored with rest.
3. The symptoms respond well to treatment with anticholinesterase drugs.

Typically, myasthenia gravis affects the bulbar innervated muscles, i.e. the extra ocular and facial muscles. Ptosis, double vision, dysarthria and dysphagia are common symptoms. Limb and neck muscle weakness may also be present. The muscle weakness is sometimes confined to the extra ocular muscles (ocular myasthenia) but more often affects multiple muscle groups (generalised myasthenia).

Severe infection, thyrotoxicosis, emotional trauma and the administration of drugs that block neuromuscular transmission, e.g. gentamycin, streptomycin, etc., may precipitate a myasthenic crisis (sudden severe muscle weakness and respiratory failure). Myasthenic crisis is a major life-threatening emergency that requires urgent treatment in a specialist intensive care unit. Treatment of the precipitating illness, respiratory support, plasma exchange and corticosteroids are the mainstay to manage a myasthenic crisis.

Diagnosis
Detection of acetylcholine receptor (AChR) antibodies and EMG studies are necessary for confirmation of the diagnosis. AChR antibodies are detectable in the serum in 90% of patients with generalised myasthenia and in 70% of patients with the localised form of the disease.

Recording of the EMG during repetitive nerve stimulation typically shows progressive decrement of the compound motor action potential. Single fibre EMG demonstrates an abnormal jitter. (Jitter is the random variability in the interval between two successive action potentials recorded from the same muscle fibre.) The diagnostic investigation of a patient with suspected myasthenia gravis should also include CT scan of the thorax to exclude or confirm the presence of a thymoma.

Treatment

Most patients respond well to treatment with anticholinesterase inhibitors, such as pyridostigmine. In refractory cases immunosuppressive treatment, e.g. corticosteroids or azathioprine, is indicated. Severe, life-threatening symptoms (myasthenic crisis) require plasma exchange or treatment with intravenous immunoglobulin. Thymectomy often results in long periods of symptomatic improvement.

The diagnosis and treatment of muscles diseases

Muscle diseases should be distinguished from chronic polyneuropathies and progressive muscular atrophy (see motor neurone disease). Although the history, the distribution of muscle weakness, the absence of sensory signs and the preservation of the tendon reflexes are helpful, laboratory investigations are usually required for the confirmation the diagnosis. Muscle imaging, electrophysiological studies, muscle biopsy and genetic tests are the main investigations.

Muscle imaging is an important part of the diagnostic workup of muscle disease. Valuable information can be obtained from CT scans and ultrasound, but MRI scans have a better resolution and are the preferred investigation. Brain imaging provides information on the pattern and extent of the muscle involvement, the disease severity (degree of muscle atrophy, the connective tissue changes and degree of replacement of muscle by fatty tissue). It is also useful for identifying the best site for muscle biopsy.

Nerve conduction studies and electromyography (EMG), including single fibre EMG, are useful for excluding other disorders, such as chronic polyneuropathies and motor neurone disease. However, confirmation of the definitive diagnosis of a myopathy and its type in most cases requires a muscle biopsy. Genetic testing is an essential part of the diagnostic workup of the hereditary myopathies.

Management

The aims of muscle disease management:

1. To reverse or reduce the disabling effects of the muscle weakness, when possible.
2. To enable the patient to maintain his functional abilities through effective rehabilitation and the provision of aids and equipment.
3. To treat the neurological impairments, such as dysphagia, dysarthria, etc.
4. To prevent and treat the complications of muscle weakness, e.g. contractures, scoliosis.
5. To provide psychological and practical support for the patient and his family, including genetic counselling.
6. Planning of terminal care in cases of end-stage muscle disease is also an important aspect of the management.

CHAPTER 13

THE NEUROLOGICAL COMPLICATIONS OF SYSTEMIC DISEASES AND DRUGS

Nervous system dysfunction may result from cardiovascular disease; systemic infections; autoimmune disease; metabolic, endocrine and haematological disorders; nutritional deficiencies; and malignant tumours. Neurological complications can also result from the toxicity of many different drugs.

The main complications of cardiovascular disease are stroke, hypertensive encephalopathy and eclampsia. These are discussed in Chapter 4. Chapter 6 deals with the neurological disorders due to systemic infections. As mentioned in Chapter 10, malignant tumours affect the nervous system by causing paraneoplastic non-metastatic syndromes, e.g. cerebellar degeneration or peripheral neuropathy, or by secondary metastatic spread to the brain and spinal cord. Haematological disorders, e.g. sickle cell disease, polycythaemia rubra vera and clotting disorders, often cause stroke and subdural haematomas. The most common metabolic disease that causes neurological complications is diabetes mellitus.

Diabetes mellitus

Diabetes mellitus causes acute and many chronic neurological complications including multi-infarct dementia due to small vessel disease, increased risk of stroke, metabolic encephalopathy due to ketoacidosis, and peripheral nervous system (PNS) disorders. The frequency of these complications correlates with the duration of diabetes and the quality of glycaemic control. Diabetics also have a high incidence of entrapment neuropathies, such as carpal tunnel and cubital tunnel syndromes, and chronic demyelinating inflammatory polyradiculoneuropathy.

The main acute neurological complications of diabetes mellitus result from either hyperglycaemia or hypoglycaemia. Hyperglycaemia associated with diabetic ketoacidosis causes mental confusion, stupor and coma. The symptoms are usually precipitated by infection, poor compliance with the treatment of diabetes, consumption of large amounts of alcohol, or the use of certain drugs, such as corticosteroids, thiazide diuretics and propranolol.

The brain is very sensitive to hypoglycaemia, as it needs half the amount of glucose utilised by the whole body. Consequently, recurrent severe hypoglycaemia often causes severe brain injury.

Mild hypoglycaemia is very common in patients on insulin treatment. It is often asymptomatic, but it can also cause mental confusion, erratic behaviour and poor mental concentration. The initial symptoms of severe hypoglycaemia are those of autonomic dysfunction, e.g. sweating, tremor and palpitations. These are usually followed by mental confusion, drowsiness and epileptic seizures. If the hypoglycaemia is not quickly reversed, the patient may become comatose. Severe prolonged hypoglycaemia may also cause irreversible brain death. Chronic frequently recurrent hypoglycaemia can result in cognitive impairment due to chronic encephalopathy.

The diabetic PNS disorders are predominantly sensory symmetrical polyneuropathy (or less often motor symmetrical polyneuropathy), symmetrical polyneuropathy, mononeuropathies, multiple mononeuropathies (mononeuritis multiplex), autonomic neuropathy, radiculopathies and diabetic amyotrophy. Isolated cranial nerve palsies, especially of the oculomotor nerve, may also occur. These complications are very common and their incidence correlates with the duration of the disease and quality of diabetic control.

Symmetrical sensory polyneuropathy (SSPN)
SSPN is the most common form of peripheral neuropathy in diabetics. It accounts for more than half the PNS complications of diabetes mellitus. In some cases, a mild sensory polyneuropathy develops in patients with glucose intolerance (i.e. the pre-diabetic stage). This condition is known

as hyperglycaemic neuropathy. It is quickly reversible with good glycaemic control.

In the early stage, SSPN is usually asymptomatic. The initial clinical presentation in the symptomatic phase is with distal dysaesthesia and sensory impairment in the toes of both feet. As the neuropathy worsens, the symptoms progress proximally. A sharp, stabbing pain and electric shock-like sensations, which are more severe at night, are prominent symptoms in some cases.

Chronic severe SSPN often causes severe complications including foot ulceration due to a combination of skin sensory loss and ischaemia, Charcot joints, and sensory ataxia often resulting in an abnormal gait.

Treatment consists of controlling hyperglycaemia, lifestyle modifications and the symptomatic management of pain. The pain usually responds to tricyclic antidepressants or anticonvulsant drugs, e.g. sodium valproate.

Diabetic amyotrophy
Diabetic amyotrophy (also called proximal diabetic neuropathy, femoral neuropathy or lumbosacral plexopathy) is an acute or subacute proximal lower limb motor neuropathy. It is rare, mainly affects older people with type 2 diabetes, and its occurrence is not related to the duration of diabetes or the quality of diabetic control.

The initial presentation is severe pain in the thighs, buttocks and lower back. Severe muscle weakness and wasting develop quickly. The clinical signs are usually confined to one side, but rapidly progress to involve the other limb and spread distally. Recovery is slow and occurs over several months. The upper limb muscles are also affected in approximately a third of cases.

Systemic vasculitis

Neurological complications are common in primary systemic vasculitis, e.g. giant cell arteritis or polyarteritis nodosa, and in conditions that cause secondary systemic vasculitis, such as connective tissue disorders, hepatitis

B or inflammatory bowel disease. The main neurological complications are cerebral vasculitis, vasculitic myelopathy and peripheral neuropathies.

The clinical features of cerebral vasculitis are headaches, seizures, mental confusion, depression and various focal neurological signs. In addition, there is evidence of systemic illness, e.g. low-grade fever, night sweats, malaise, arthralgia and weight loss. The C-reactive protein and erythrocyte sedimentation rate are high. Normochromic, normocytic anaemia is common. CSF examination shows high protein and pleocytosis. Multifocal ischaemic lesions are present on the MRI brain scan. Cerebral angiography and brain biopsy may be required for confirmation of the diagnosis.

Vasculitic neuropathies result from the inflammation of the vasa nervorum (the epineurial arteries of peripheral nerves), thrombosis and ischaemia. Most frequently the patients develop multiple mononeuropathies (mononeuritis multiplex), mononeuropathies or a sensorimotor symmetrical polyneuropathy. The onset may be acute, subacute or chronic. Systemic symptoms, including fever and weight loss, are usually present.

Treatment of vasculitis is with high doses of corticosteroids and other immunosuppressive therapy, e.g. azathioprine or methotrexate.

Renal and hepatic encephalopathies

Encephalopathy is common in patients with acute or chronic end-stage renal failure. The encephalopathy becomes symptomatic usually when the glomerular filtration rate falls to less than 10% of its normal value. The initial manifestations are excessive fatigue, hyperactivity and sleep disturbances. With further deterioration of the renal function, the patient becomes confused, paranoid, and develops myoclonus and epileptic seizures. Frequently there is also evidence of a peripheral neuropathy.

Haemodialysis is also a cause of encephalopathy. The encephalopathy (or dialysis disequilibrium syndrome) results from the rapid fluid shifts and electrolyte disturbances. The symptoms usually start 24 hours after dialysis and consist of headaches, muscle cramps, mental confusion and, sometimes, seizures. They often resolve spontaneously after one or two days. Haemodialysis may also occasionally cause intracerebral bleeding.

Liver failure and portal hypertension also result in encephalopathy. The symptoms are similar to those described above. An additional typical feature is asterixis (also called the 'liver flap'). It is elicited by asking the patients to extend his arms and dorsiflex the wrist. This causes sudden flexion of the wrist.

Nutritional deficiencies

Nutritional deficiencies are caused by a poor diet or diseases that interfere with absorption of nutrients (mainly vitamins). The most common nutritional deficiencies that cause neurological disease are those of vitamin B1 (thiamine) and B12 (cobalamin). Deficiency of vitamin B3 (nicotinic acid) is rare in high-income countries, except among alcoholics. It is often combined with protein-calorie malnutrition and causes pellagra (dermatitis, diarrhoea and delirium). Thiamine deficiency causes Wernicke's encephalopathy and Korsakoff's syndrome.

Wernicke's encephalopathy and Korsakoff's syndrome

Wernicke's encephalopathy (WE) is an acute neuropsychiatric syndrome due to thiamine (vitamin B1) deficiency. It is common in alcoholics due to a combination of poor diet and the effects of alcohol on thiamine metabolism. Alcohol interferes with thiamine absorption, storage in the liver (due to alcoholic liver disease), transport across the blood-brain barrier, and utilisation by brain cells.

The main features of WE are mental confusion, impaired cognitive function, cerebellar ataxia, ophthalmoplegia, nystagmus, and conjugate gaze paralysis. Brain imaging demonstrates lesions mainly in the mammillary bodies, periaqueductal area and thalamus. Treatment is with high-dose intravenous thiamine (500 mg three times per day for 3-5 days, followed by an oral maintenance dose). Untreated, or inadequately treated, WE evolves into Korsakoff's syndrome (KS). KS is characterised by severe irreversible amnesia, disorientation, confabulations and the reduced ability to learn new material.

Vitamin B12 deficiency

Vitamin B12 deficiency usually results from malabsorption (pernicious anaemia, atrophic gastritis, Crohn's disease) or poor dietary intake, e.g. strict vegan diet, alcoholism. It causes subacute combined degeneration of the spinal cord, peripheral neuropathy, optic atrophy and cognitive dysfunction.

Subacute combined degeneration of the spinal cord (SCD)

SCD is characterised by degeneration of the posterior and lateral columns of the spinal cord resulting in sensory ataxia and spastic paraparesis. Peripheral neuropathy, visual and cognitive impairment are also present in severe cases. The onset is insidious and the disease is slowly progressive. The initial symptoms are distal paraesthesia of all limbs, leg stiffness and unsteady gait.

In the absence of a history of alcoholism, the most likely cause is pernicious anaemia, atrophic gastritis or Crohn's disease. (Vitamin B12 is absorbed in the stomach and terminal ileum.) The presence of megaloblastic anaemia is a useful diagnostic clue and suggests pernicious anaemia. The diagnosis is confirmed by measuring the serum vitamin B12 and methylmalonic acid, and the detection of serum antibodies against the gastric parietal cells and the intrinsic factor. Treatment with vitamin B12 injections is required for life.

Prescription drugs

Many drugs cause neurological complications, and drug toxicity may affect any part of the nervous system. Only a few of the most frequently used drugs are listed here.

Cognitive dysfunction: anticholinergic drugs, benzodiazepines, levodopa and dopamine agonists.

Cerebellar degeneration: anticonvulsants, especially phenytoin.

Extrapyramidal syndromes (parkinsonism, dystonia, dyskinesia): neuroleptic drugs and butyrophenones, e.g. haloperidol.

Peripheral neuropathy: amiodarone, colchicine, ethambutol, metronidazole, nitrofurantoin, isoniazid, chloroquine, phenytoin and most anticancer drugs.

Seizures: phenothiazines, monoamine oxidase inhibitors.

Myopathy: corticosteroids, statins, penicillamine, antimalarials, interferon, antiretroviral drugs (e.g. zidovudine).

The effects of alcohol and illicit drugs

Alcohol (ethanol) use and misuse is common throughout the world. Excessive and chronic consumption of alcohol often causes serious illnesses, including liver and heart disease and many neurological disorders. The brain is particularly sensitive to the effects of alcohol. These effects are due to the action of alcohol on various neurotransmitter systems.

Alcohol enhances the inhibitory action of gamma aminobutyric acid (GABA) on neurotransmission resulting in sedation, disinhibition and a feeling of relaxation. However, the GABA receptors are downregulated with chronic alcohol use and this is thought to be the cause of alcohol withdrawal symptoms.

Alcohol also reduces the excitatory glutamate central neurotransmission. This explains the attention deficits and difficulties with acquisition of new memory due to alcohol use. Chronic alcohol consumption causes upregulation of glutamate receptors, which may precipitate epileptic seizures.

Alcohol is usually used because it elevates mood and gives a sense of well-being and pleasure. This effect is due to its action on the brain's reward dopaminergic and opioid receptors of the limbic system. Downregulation of these receptors probably leads to alcohol dependency.

Heavy chronic alcohol consumption causes severe brain atrophy, especially of the frontal lobes, the hippocampus and cerebellum. The neurological complications result from direct alcohol toxicity and from nutritional deficiencies. Older subjects and adolescents are more vulnerable to the toxic effects of alcohol. However, there is no agreement on the amount of alcohol that is considered safe. In the UK at present, the maximum safe amount of alcohol is considered 14 units per week spread over 3 or 4 days. (A unit of alcohol is defined as 8 grams of pure alcohol. This is approximately equivalent to half a pint of beer of average strength or a small glass of low strength wine.) The safe amount is less for women and thin individuals. It is also considerably less for pregnant women and for people with liver disease, brain injury or mental health disorders.

The neurological effects of acute alcohol intoxication

The main effects of acute alcohol intoxication are impairment of motor coordination, sensory perception and cognitive function. Drowsiness, disinhibition, jocularity or aggressive behaviour may also occur. There are large variations between individuals in the alcohol blood concentration that results in acute intoxication. Tolerance to alcohol, the amount drunk and the rate of rise in alcohol blood levels appear to be important factors. (Tolerance to alcohol is usually associated with previous frequent use and is also mediated by genetic factors.) In most individuals, alcohol blood levels of 30-65 ml/dl result in acute toxicity.

The neurological complications of excessive chronic alcohol use

Chronic heavy alcohol consumption results in numerous serious neurological complications. These include painful peripheral neuropathy, cerebellar degeneration, dementia, Wernicke's encephalopathy, myopathy, increased stroke risk, and epilepsy. Traumatic brain injury and chronic subdural haematomas due to frequent falls are common in alcoholics. Excessive alcohol consumption during pregnancy may cause foetal neurodevelopmental abnormalities.

Delirium tremens

Sudden reduction or complete withdrawal of alcohol after chronic heavy drinking often results in alcohol withdrawal syndromes. Delirium tremens is the most serious of these disorders. It is potentially life-threatening.

Delirium tremens is characterised by severe acute mental confusion, hallucinations and symptoms of sympathetic overactivity (such as tachycardia, cardiac arrhythmias, tremor, excessive sweating and hyperpyrexia).

The management of severe cases of delirium tremens should be carried out in an intensive care unit. Sedation with a benzodiazepine and haloperidol, correction of any metabolic and electrolyte abnormalities, and general life support measures are the mainstay of the initial treatment. Severe cases have a high mortality rate, and death is often due to severe cardiac arrhythmias.

Alcohol-drug interactions
Alcohol also interacts with numerous drugs, including many CNS-active drugs. Of the drugs used in neurological disorders, perhaps the most clinically important interactions are with the antiepileptic drugs. Alcohol induces liver enzymes and reduces the blood concentrations of carbamazepine and phenytoin. It also increases the sedative and hypotensive effects of sedative and hypnotic drugs, and most antidepressants.

The effects of illicit drugs
Illicit recreational drugs, such as cannabis, heroin, cocaine and methamphetamine, may cause various neuropsychiatric disorders including severe headaches, seizures, stroke, parkinsonism, depression and acute psychosis. Chronic use can also result in cognitive impairment. A sudden surge in blood pressure, cardiac arrhythmias, focal or segmental vasospasm, emboli from cardiac vegetations, and neuronal degeneration are possible mechanisms.

CHAPTER 14

TRAUMA OF THE NERVOUS SYSTEM

Blunt brain injuries, and to a less extent spinal cord and peripheral nerve injuries, are common and often result in significant long-term disability. Road traffic accidents, falls, and assault are the main causes. Alcohol intoxication is often a contributing factor. Penetrating gunshot and blast injuries are a common cause of CNS trauma in military combat.

Although this chapter deals with traumatic brain injury that is acquired after childhood, infants who survive brain injury sustained in the perinatal period causing cerebral palsy (CP) invariably continue to have neurological symptoms, e.g. epilepsy, spasticity, throughout their adult life and are often referred to neurology clinics. Therefore, a brief description of CP is included in this chapter.

Traumatic brain injury

Traumatic brain injury (TBI) is defined as disruption of the brain's structure and/or function caused by the impact of an external mechanical force and occurring immediately after the trauma. The disruption of brain function includes all or any of the following: loss of consciousness, altered mental state (e.g. confusion, disorientation), post-traumatic amnesia and focal neurological deficits.

TBI is a common cause of death and disability. The incidence of TBI in most European countries varies between 200 and 250 cases per 100,000 of the population per year. The peak incidence of TBI is bimodal affecting young adults (mostly men) and older people.

Pathology of TBI

TBI occurs when a strong blow to the head results in a fast head movement, which ceases abruptly as the head comes into contact with a hard object, e.g. the ground. This acceleration-deceleration force generates rotational forces and shearing stresses that cause diffuse axonal injuries, and compression of neural tissues and blood vessels. Other pathological changes are contusions, lacerations and haemorrhages.

The primary effects of brain injury, i.e. the direct effects of the mechanical force, are two types: focal and diffuse. The focal injuries are skull fractures, contusions, lacerations and haematomas. The contusions (bruising of tissue) typically occur in the inferior aspects and poles of the frontal lobes and the inferior aspects of the temporal lobes. Trauma to the front of the head frequently causes contusions on the side of the impact (coup contusions). By contrast, a strike to the back of the head, as a rule, results in contusions on the frontal lobes, i.e. the side opposite to the head trauma (counter coup contusions). When the head is struck on the side, the patient may have either coup or counter coup contusions.

The primary diffuse effects of TBI is diffuse axonal injury with subsequent Wallerian degeneration, and metabolic and neurotransmitter dysfunction. Cytotoxic cerebral oedema, hypoxia, hypotension, ischaemia and hyperglycaemia lead to secondary brain damage.

Cerebral cytotoxic oedema is an important cause of secondary brain injury. In contrast to vasogenic oedema (which results from the increased permeability of the vascular endothelium), cytotoxic oedema is due to the effects of hypoxia and ischaemia. It causes fluid shift from the extracellular to the intracellular space. Massive cerebral oedema often increases the intracranial pressure. Severely raised intracranial pressure may cause displacement of brain structures and herniation through the tentorium or the foramen magnum.

The clinical features of TBI

The clinical features of TBI mainly depend on the severity of the injury. The most widely used method for grading the severity of TBI is the modified Glasgow Coma Scale (GCS). As mentioned in Chapter 3, the GCS measures the patient's eye opening, and motor and verbal responses. A score of 13 to 14 on the GCS indicates mild TBI. Moderately severe and severe TBI are defined as a score of 9-12 and 8 or less, respectively.

Mild TBI (concussion) is the most frequent form of brain injury. The patient complains of headaches, dizziness, unsteady gait and blurred vision. In mild cases there is no loss of consciousness. The patient has a very brief post-traumatic amnesia lasting less than 30 minutes and complete resolution of the symptoms occurs in less than 24 hours. Severe concussion is characterised by loss of consciousness for 1 minute or more and amnesia lasting more than 24 hours. Transient blindness or transient paraplegia may occur in cases of severe concussion. In some cases these symptoms persist for weeks or months. In addition, many patients develop irritability, fatigue, poor mental concentration, intolerance of noise, anxiety and depression. Sleep disturbances, e.g. insomnia, excessive sleep and parasomnias, are also common.

Patients with severe and moderately severe TBI present with deep coma and autonomic nervous system dysfunction, including tachycardia, tachypnoea, hypertension and profuse sweating. The autonomic dysfunction is usually transient. Its persistence is associated with poor clinical outcomes.

The course of TBI in patients with severe or moderately severe injuries is variable. Approximately 20-30% of these patients die in the first 4 weeks despite specialist medical care. However, in most cases the autonomic dysfunction stabilises and gradual recovery starts within days or weeks. Few patients develop the permanent vegetative state (PVS). (PVS is described in Chapter 3.)

Recovery usually occurs in the following sequence: After a period in deep coma, the patient starts to intermittently open his eyes, move his limbs and vocalise for a short period, and then lapses again into coma. These periods of improved level of consciousness progressively lengthen. He then regains consciousness but remains confused. The confusional state is followed by post-traumatic amnesia. In parallel with these changes, there is also gradual improvement in the focal neurological deficits. However, complete neurological and functional recovery is rare. Most patients with severe TBI continue to have long-term physical disability, cognitive impairment and personality change.

Skull fractures are a common complication of TBI. The clinical effects of basal skull fractures are particularly significant. These fractures often cause cranial nerve injuries, usually the optic, olfactory, trigeminal and the oculomotor nerves. Other effects of basal skull fractures are injuries to the pituitary gland, dural tears resulting in otorrhoea and rhinorrhoea due to CSF leak, and laceration of the intracavernous portion of the internal carotid artery, and the formation a carotidocavernous fistula and pulsating exophthalmos. Skull fractures also increase the risk of CNS infections (meningitis, brain abscess). Frequently, fractures of the cribriform plate of the ethmoid bone cause permanent anosmia.

Diagnosis
The investigation of choice for patients presenting with moderately severe or severe TBI is CT head scans. However, their diagnostic value in mild TBI is limited except when there is loss of consciousness for more than five minutes, seizures, focal neurological signs or long periods of post-injury mental confusion or disorientation. Brain imaging is also indicated in patients with depressed skull fractures, basal skull fractures or penetrating head injuries. TBI in the context of alcohol intoxication, irrespective of its severity, is also an indication for brain imaging.

Treatment
Patients with severe and moderately severe TBI are best managed in a specialist neurocritical care unit. The resuscitation of these patients should start at the scene of the accident. The prompt correction of hypoxia, hypotension, hyperglycaemia and hyponatraemia minimise the risk of secondary brain injury and improve the clinical outcomes. Tracheal intubation and ventilation is necessary in most cases.

Monitoring of the intracranial pressure is an essential aspect of the management of severe TBI. Severe cerebral oedema requires treatment with osmotic agents (mannitol or hypertonic saline). Decompressive craniectomy is indicated if the conservative medical treatment fails.

The management in the post-acute phase consists of symptom-specific treatment (e.g. seizures, spasticity, etc.) and rehabilitation.

The long-term consequences of TBI

Severe and moderately severe TBI result in many complications including epilepsy, endocrine dysfunction, post-concussional syndrome, chronic encephalopathy, parkinsonism and Korsakoff's psychosis.

Post-traumatic epilepsy

Epilepsy occurs in approximately 5% of patients with blunt TBI and in 50% of patients with penetrating TBI. The first seizure can occur any time after the injury, but usually in the first 6 months.

Hypothalamic-pituitary dysfunction

The main endocrine abnormalities in the acute phase of TBI (usually defined as the first two weeks post-injury) are the syndrome of inappropriate antidiuretic hormone secretion and diabetes insipidus. They are usually transient, and complete recovery occurs in most cases in the first six months post-injury. Panhypopituitarism is also common.

Panhypopituitarism may occur any time during the first year after TBI. Hypogonadism and hyperprolactinaemia occur in the acute phase and are considered to be an adaptive response to the injury. The cause of hypopituitarism is not fully understood. The direct effect of the trauma, hypoxia and ischaemia are possible mechanisms. Hypopituitarism is associated with poor neurological and functional recovery. Therefore, it is essential to monitor the pituitary function periodically in the first year of TBI, especially when the neurological and functional recovery is slower or less than expected.

The post-concussional syndrome

The behavioural, cognitive and emotional symptoms of concussion completely resolve within 1 or 2 weeks in more than 80% of patients. The persistence of these symptoms for 6 weeks or longer is known as the post-concussional syndrome (PCS). Old age, female gender, history of mental illness and a low socio-economic status increase the risk of developing the PCS.

The management of the PCS consists of counselling, cognitive rehabilitation, medical treatment of symptoms (e.g. depression, anxiety, insomnia), and the gradual return to physical activity and work. The prognosis for recovery is variable. Lack of social support and ongoing litigation for compensation are often associated with poor recovery.

Chronic traumatic encephalopathy

Repeated concussion may cause chronic traumatic encephalopathy (CTE). CTE is known to occur in professional boxers and those who play contact sports, such as American football and soccer. The disorder is characterised by progressive widespread loss of cortical and subcortical neurons, and neurofibrillary tangles (especially in the frontal and temporal lobes).

The symptoms usually manifest decades after the last trauma. Irritability, personality change, emotional lability, poor memory and disinhibition are frequently the initial symptoms. As the disease progresses, the symptoms of cognitive impairment become more severe and the patient develops signs of parkinsonism. Dementia is a late feature of the disease. Brain imaging demonstrates diffuse brain atrophy.

The social consequences of TBI

Cognitive deficits and behavioural changes are common after TBI irrespective of the severity of the injury. They result in poor social functioning. Patients are often unable to maintain existing family relationships or develop new personal relationships. The cognitive impairment and poor social skills frequently result in unemployment and, in some cases, they may also lead to criminality.

Prognosis

The mortality rate of patients with severe or moderately severe TBI is high. Approximately 50% of those with GCS score less than 8, and 30% of patients with a score less than 13 die in the first few weeks after the injury.

The strongest predictors of poor prognosis are a low GCS score on admission, penetrating injuries, old age, female gender, midline shift of brain structures on CT scan, and subdural haematoma. These patients usually have less functional recovery and are more likely to need long-term institutional care.

Cerebral palsy

Cerebral palsy (CP) is a disorder of brain development that results from traumatic brain injury or hypoxic-ischaemic damage in the perinatal period. The disorder primarily affects the motor system and may or may not cause other neurological deficits. Although the underlying pathology in CP is non-progressive, the disability associated with the disease may worsen over time.

The overall incidence of CP in Western Europe is approximately less than 3 cases per 1000 live births. Prematurity, a low birth weight and a low socio-economic status of the child's parents appear to be significant risk factors for developing CP in full term (but not premature) infants. The brain damage in CP is caused by different mechanisms. Neonatal asphyxia is a common aetiological factor. Other causes include perinatal traumatic brain injury (e.g. as a result of forceps delivery), intra-uterine (foetal) infections and poorly controlled maternal epilepsy during pregnancy.

Different classifications of CP have been proposed. The most widely accepted one identifies four main types of CP. These are spastic, athetoid, ataxic, and mixed CP. The spastic type is further subdivided into spastic hemiplegia, diplegia (all limbs are involved, but the legs are more affected than the arms), double hemiplegia, and tetraplegia or total body involvement.

Clinical presentation

Because myelination of the pyramidal tract is not complete until the age of 18-24 months, the neurological signs of its dysfunction during this period are often subtle. The infant with CP may, therefore, appear normal at birth and the first indication of the disease is often noticed a few weeks or months later. Early signs include increased or reduced muscle tone, asymmetry of posture or movements, abnormalities of postural and righting reflexes, or persistence of primitive reflexes (such the rooting reflex). Delay in the developmental milestones is another common, but non-specific, feature. Epilepsy, intellectual and sensory deficits are common, especially in the severe types of CP such as spastic tetraplegia.

CP in adults

The majority of children with CP survive into adulthood with over 80% attaining at least middle age. The severity of the cognitive and motor deficits is important in determining life expectancy. However, even in the presence of marked cognitive impairments, two-thirds of subjects reach the age of 35 years. A significant proportion of adults with CP will gradually lose some of their functional independence with mobility and activities of daily living in a relatively short time. This deterioration occurs in a third of cases over a five-year period and it is most likely to occur in the more severely affected individuals. Adults with CP are often referred to neurology clinics for the management of epilepsy, poor mobility, spasticity, progressive dysarthria and increasing physical dependency.

Disorders of mobility are common. Severe hypotonia and/or poor balance and posture may result in difficulties with mobility and ambulation in patients with the athetoid and ataxic forms of CP. However, spasticity is by far the most common cause of locomotor disability in patients with this disorder. It leads to characteristic abnormalities of gait including scissoring, crouch gait and equinus gait. The locomotor disability in young adults with athetoid CP may be aggravated by the development of cervical myelopathy and/or radiculopathy, presumably due to excessive neck movements.

Dysarthria is also common and may be the result of spasticity, muscle weakness or the poor muscle coordination due to ataxia or orofacial dyskinesia. In severe cases, verbal communication becomes difficult or impossible. This often prevents affected individuals from making friendships, pursuing leisure activities or taking employment, and may lead to social isolation and depression.

Prognosis

Those with tetraplegia (total body involvement) have the highest incidence of intellectual deficits, epilepsy and deafness among patients with CP. This form of the disease generally carries a poor prognosis, both for long-term survival and for functional independence. Similarly, choreoathetoid CP is usually associated with severe disability and responds less favourably to therapeutic interventions.

Spinal cord injuries

Spinal cord injuries (SCI) are 10 times less common than TBI. They are most frequently caused by road traffic accidents, falls from height, sports injury (e.g. rugby, horse riding, diving into shallow water) and assault. Spinal injuries should always be suspected in patients with severe TBI. A third of patients with severe TBI caused by road traffic accidents also have a spinal injury.

Pathology

More than half the SCI affect the cervical spine and another 30-35% involve the thoracic spine. Pure SCIs are rare. In most cases, there is also fracture-dislocation or dislocation of one or more vertebrae and ligaments damage. The injury causes destruction of the grey and white matter and haemorrhages in the spinal cord with subsequent tissue necrosis, gliosis and cavity formation. These changes are maximal at the level of the injury, and two or three segments above and below it.

Clinical features

The clinical features depend on the level and severity of the SCI. Tetraplegia results from C4-C5 cervical lesions, and paraplegia results from thoracic lesions. The type of injury (fracture-dislocation, dislocation without a fracture, etc.) and the level of the SCI are best confirmed with MRI scans.

The initial phase of SCI is characterised by a 'spinal shock'. Spinal shock is believed to be due to the sudden loss of the supra segmental control on the spinal neuronal circuits. It is characterised by flaccid paralysis and sensory loss below the level of the lesion, areflexia, autonomic system dysfunction, and an atonic bladder and bowel. Gastroparesis and ileus may also be present. The phase of spinal shock usually lasts a few weeks and is followed by spastic paraplegia or tetraplegia with sensory loss to the level of the injury, and bowel and bladder dysfunction. Detrusor-sphincter dyssynergia (see Chapter 3 for details) is a common complication.

Respiratory insufficiency is common in patients with high SCI. It usually results from partial paralysis of the diaphragm or weak intercostal muscles. Other causes are sputum retention due to the inability to cough, and lung contusions or pneumothorax sustained during the initial trauma.

In the period that follows the spinal shock patients with cervical or high thoracic (above D6) lesions become susceptible to a syndrome, known as autonomic dysreflexia, caused by the overactivity of the sympathetic nervous system.

Autonomic dysreflexia is usually precipitated by urinary retention, infections, detrusor-sphincter dyssynergia, faecal impaction, infected pressure sores, and bladder calculi. The patient complains of severe throbbing headaches and profuse sweating. The blood pressure is very high and there is often red skin discolouration above the level of the lesion due to vasodilatation. Autonomic dysreflexia may cause intracerebral or subarachnoid haemorrhage unless promptly treated.

Treatment
The initial management of severe SCI consists of the reduction of the vertebral dislocation by skeleton traction, immobilisation or surgical decompression, the treatment of symptoms (hypotension, respiratory insufficiency, pain, depression, etc.), prevention of the complications of immobility (deep vein thrombosis, skin pressure sores and bladder calculi), the maintenance of hydration and nutrition, bladder and bowel training, and rehabilitation.

The prompt treatment of autonomic dysreflexia is of paramount importance. It consists of the management of the precipitating factor and the administration of sublingual nifedipine (5-10 mg).

Prognosis

The prognosis of SCI depends mainly on the severity of the injury (i.e. complete or incomplete) and the level of the lesion. Complete cervical cord lesions have the worst prognosis for survival in the first year after the SCI, life expectancy and functional recovery. Other poor prognostic factors are old age, low socio-economic status, substance abuse and psychiatric co-morbidity.

The mortality rate in the early period after SCI is highest in patients with injuries above C4 and is mainly due to respiratory failure. Other causes of death in the acute phase are shock, infections and ileus. The mortality rate reduces significantly after the first 3 months of SCI; more than 80% of patients survive 10 years or more.

Peripheral nervous system injuries

Upper limb nerve injuries

The peripheral nerves of the upper limbs are more vulnerable to trauma compared to those in the lower limbs. Fractures of the neck of the humerus or a shoulder dislocation may cause injury to the axillary nerve resulting in weakness and wasting of the deltoid muscle. Fractures of the shaft of the humerus often cause radial nerve injury. This causes weakness of the triceps muscle and the finger extensors, and loss of the triceps and supinator tendon reflexes. Injury to the ulnar and median nerves occurs as a direct trauma to the elbow or wrist, respectively.

The most serious upper limb nerve injury is brachial plexus avulsion. It most frequently affects the upper trunk (Erb-Duchenne paralysis) or the lower trunk (Klumpke's paralysis).

The upper trunk of the brachial plexus is most frequently injured as a result of motorcycle accidents or during forceps delivery of newborn babies. The upper trunk consists of C5 and C6 nerve roots. It innervates the deltoid, infraspinatus, supraspinatus, biceps and brachioradialis muscles. In addition to pain around the shoulder and in the proximal part of the arm, injury to these nerve roots causes weakness of shoulder abduction and elbow flexion, and wasting of the deltoid, infraspinatus, supraspinatus, biceps brachii and brachioradialis muscles. The biceps tendon reflex is depressed or absent.

Injury of the lower trunk of the brachial plexus (C8 and D1) is less common and usually results from forceful pulling on the outstretched arm, e.g. when a person holds onto an object above his head during a fall from height. (The most common lesions of the lower brachial plexus trunk are non-traumatic, and include carcinoma of the lung apex and metastases from breast carcinoma.) This division of the brachial plexus innervates the small muscles of the hands and the finger flexors and extensors. Its injury causes wasting and weakness of the hand muscles and the fingers flexors and extensors, impaired skin sensation on the medial aspect of the forearm and loss of the finger jerk.

Lower limb nerve injuries
Trauma of the peripheral nerves of the lower limbs is rare. The most common injury is compression of the peroneal nerve at the head of the fibula resulting in foot drop usually without sensory loss. The injury is typically due to sitting with the legs crossed for long periods. (More frequently, the causes of foot drop due to peroneal nerve lesions are non-traumatic and include diabetes mellitus and connective tissue disease.)

The obturator nerve in the pelvis may be damaged during forceps delivery. Injury to this nerve causes pain in the anterior aspect of the thigh, weakness of hip adduction and loss of the adductor reflex. Usually there is no sensory loss.

Fractures of the pelvis or the top part of the femur that involve the acetabulum often cause injury to the femoral nerve. The patient presents with weakness of hip flexion, knee extension and absent knee jerk. Skin sensation is reduced or absent on the antero-medial aspect of the thigh and the whole leg to the medial malleolus.

CHAPTER 15

NEUROREHABILITATION

Neurological disorders often cause severe long-term functional disability. The patient's mobility, independence with personal care and other activities of daily living, and his ability to pursue employment and leisure activities can all be affected. Complete recovery after the specific drug treatment of the underlying illness is relatively rare and most patients will require rehabilitation to regain their functional independence.

Rehabilitation is a coordinated goal-directed process of therapy interventions that aims to reverse the loss of functional abilities due to disease or injury, or to enhance the patient's residual functional abilities.

The process of rehabilitation
Effective rehabilitation is a coordinated multidisciplinary activity. Although individual therapy interventions are important for promoting recovery, it is generally recognised that the quality of the overall rehabilitation programme is what determines the final functional outcomes for the patient. In addition to delivering the appropriate remedial therapies, the rehabilitation programme should aim to utilise the patient's positive personal attributes and take into account the physical environment to which he will return following discharge from hospital. It should also recognise the potential long-term benefits of enabling him to maintain contact with his social network.

The rehabilitation programme should be based on explicitly agreed treatment goals. The process of rehabilitation starts with an assessment of the patient's impairments, the resulting limitations in functional activities (i.e. the disabilities) and their impact on social participation. It is also important to know about the patient's personal attributes and the physical environmental and social factors that might act as assets or barriers to successful rehabilitation, and the patient's ability to maintain functional independence after discharge from hospital. This assessment is then used for setting the treatment goals and also as a baseline for monitoring the patient's response to the rehabilitation programme.

Rehabilitation is an educational process and it is important to explain to the patients the common features of their neurological disorder, how these might affect them and the best way to overcome the difficulties arising from them. The rehabilitation team should monitor the patient's progress and review the therapy plan periodically, usually once or twice a week. The team, together with the patient and his family, should also start early to plan the patient's discharge from hospital and to arrange the post-discharge follow-up and support in the community.

Assessment of the impairments and their consequences
The main physical impairments caused by neurological diseases are muscle weakness, reduction or loss of skin sensation, visual field deficits, dysphagia, dysphasia, dysarthria, dyspraxia, unilateral hemispatial neglect, poor balance and impairment of cognitive function. The methods of assessment and treatment of these impairments are described in Chapter 2.

It is important that every member of the rehabilitation team, irrespective of their speciality, has a good working knowledge of these symptoms and their possible effects on the patient's health and functional abilities. This is because the successful management of most of these impairments and their functional consequences usually requires input from different members of staff, and the contribution of each of them should be consistent and in accordance with the agreed overall therapy plan. For example, if a decision to manage unilateral hemispatial neglect with impairment training (rather than task-specific training) is made, then all team members should adopt the same strategy in all their dealings with the patient. For instance, the patient should be approached from the affected side and visual, tactile or auditory cues are used to direct his attention to the neglected hemispace when given medication by the nurse, during physiotherapy, or while undergoing training for independence with washing and dressing by the occupational therapist. Even the patient's family members and visitors should be encouraged to adopt the same approach in order to reinforce the treatment strategy.

Setting of the rehabilitation goals

A coordinated and goal-directed teamwork is the corner stone of rehabilitation. A well-organised multidisciplinary team (MDT) has unity of purpose, avoids duplication of effort by individual team members, delivers organised care (rather than random treatments) and focuses on improving the patient's functional abilities. Setting of the treatment goals is central to effective teamwork. It helps to direct the MDT activity, to motivate the patient and staff, and to enable a meaningful monitoring of the patient's improvement (or deterioration) over time against expected recovery milestones.

Treatment goals are the functional and social outcomes desired by the patient and expected to result from the rehabilitation process. They should not be confused with therapy goals, which are the actions required to direct the therapeutic and other rehabilitation interventions. For example, the treatment goal of a hemiplegic patient may involve being able to walk short distances indoors by the time they are discharged from hospital. The therapy goals relevant to this could include a series of actions of progressively increasing complexity, such as training the patient to regain his balance in sitting and standing, then to stand and practice stepping with the therapists, and then to walk on the ward with assistance, and subsequently with supervision only, etc.

The process of setting appropriate treatment goals is complex. The MDT needs to analyse the patient's impairments and their functional consequences for the patient and his carers, and to have a good knowledge of the likely course and prognosis of the underlying disease. In order to set realistic treatment goals, it is also important to consider the patient's previous level of functioning, co-morbidities and general health, and to ascertain the patient's wishes.

The patient's cooperation and motivation for a given treatment goal is likely to be influenced by his personal interest in that objective, i.e. the desired outcome of treatment, and the effort required to achieve it. The expectations of the MDT (which are usually based on their perception of the patient's needs) should not be the sole basis for setting the treatment goals because what is important to the professional staff might not be important to the patient. Therapy goals should, therefore, be negotiated and not imposed.

The acronym SMART goals (which refers to sensible, measurable, achievable, relevant and time-limited) was coined as a description of a properly set treatment goal. A sensible goal is a realistic one that takes into account the severity of the patient's impairments and previous functional abilities. It is neither too ambitious, nor too easy and is likely to be achieved with the appropriate therapeutic intervention and effort by the patient. Goal setting should also be a dynamic process because patients' needs (and their perceptions of needs) and wishes may change over time.

The aims and objectives of rehabilitation
The therapy and other rehabilitation interventions should aim:

1. To reduce the disability by managing the impairments and, through independence training, to compensate for the effects of loss of function, and to enable the acquisition of new functional skills.
2. To mitigate the impact of residual disability by the use of technology and environmental adaptations.
3. To optimise the patient's functional abilities at crisis points, e.g. sudden functional deterioration after an acute infection or a fall.
4. To prevent or treat the complications of the underlying disease, such as severe muscle spasticity, malnutrition secondary to dysphagia, etc.

The therapy interventions
Several mechanisms mediate the functional recovery after brain damage. These mechanisms are enhanced by goal-directed, task-specific training

and are maintained by reinforcement, i.e. task repetition. The acquisition of new motor and cognitive skills during rehabilitation is, therefore, influenced by the treatment intensity and the way the treatment is delivered (e.g. passive stimulation versus task-specific therapy). Although treatment is typically delivered in time-limited therapy sessions, it is important to emphasise that it should be continued on the ward by the nursing and other staff to enable further practice and consolidation of the newly acquired skills. This then facilitates the task-specific improvements in motor and other functions are incorporated into the patient's activities of daily living.

Choosing the method of the remedial therapy intervention should be individualised. For example, different treatment approaches that utilise muscle stretching and strengthening exercises, and training to improve alignment of body parts, mobility and gait, e.g. the neurodevelopmental (Bobath) method, and the proprioceptive neuromuscular facilitation technique have been advocated. However, in practice, rarely one method of physiotherapy is used exclusively and, as a rule, the different therapy methods or some of the component parts of these methods are utilised in combination when treating the same patient. Therefore, an eclectic approach that is tailored to suit the patient's rehabilitation goals is probably sufficient in most cases.

Review of the patient's response to rehabilitation
The purpose of rehabilitation is to help patients recover lost function or to develop new skills that compensate for the functional loss. Another important purpose is to facilitate the patient's emotional adjustment to the resulting residual disability and its impact on social participation and quality of life. Rehabilitation is considered successful when it enables the patient to achieve functional independence in mobility and activities of daily living, and to resume previous family and social roles, including return to gainful employment and leisure activities. Therefore, monitoring of the patient's response to rehabilitation should be based on clear functional outcome measures.

In routine clinical practice, the use of a goal attainment scale and a simple global functional scale, e.g. the Barthel index of activities of daily living, is usually sufficient. Goal attainment scales are particularly valuable because they can be adapted to the goals of the individual patient (rather than the perception of the patient's carers and the rehabilitation professionals). When seemingly realistic goals are not met, an attempt should be made to establish and rectify the cause of this failure. Common barriers to effective rehabilitation include anxiety and depression, and subclinical intercurrent illness (such as asymptomatic urinary tract infections).

Planning discharge from hospital

Most patients wish to live at home after the initial episode of care in hospital. Enabling patients to return to live in their own homes is a worthwhile aim of rehabilitation and should be pursued, whenever possible. Returning to live at home has several benefits. It helps to preserve the patients' self-identity in the face of poor health, loss of social roles and dependency. It also gives disabled individuals a sense of autonomy and control of their own affairs, and possibly motivates them to maintain their functional abilities. However, these advantages need to be weighed carefully against the possible risks of an unsafe home discharge. In addition to this risk assessment, due consideration should be given to the need for adaptations to the patient's home environment, the provision of therapy after discharge, if needed, and the practical and emotional support for patients and their carers.

The timely discharge of the patient from hospital is particularly important. Prolonged and unnecessary hospitalisation fosters functional dependency and may expose the patient to health risks, such as hospital-acquired infections. Similarly, premature discharge, especially in the absence of adequate formal and informal social support and community rehabilitation services, may lead to a loss of the functional skills that were acquired during the in-patient rehabilitation, and may trigger avoidable readmission to hospital or transfer to long-term institutional care.

There is a large variation between individuals in the degree of functional independence they need to achieve before they are fit for discharge from hospital. Nonetheless, adequate cognitive function, especially a reasonably good memory and safety judgement, and some independence with mobility and the ability to communicate with others effectively (e.g. to summon help in an emergency) are essential for patients who intend to live alone (at least for some part of the day) after they leave hospital. The use of arbitrarily chosen criteria, such as the length of hospital stay or a predetermined score on the Barthel index of activities of daily living, is usually unhelpful. Consequently, the timing of discharge from hospital should be considered on a case-by-case basis rather than based on such arbitrary criteria.

When planning the patient's discharge from hospital, the MDT should take into account the wishes of the patient and his family, the severity of functional dependency, the suitability and safety of the environment in which the patient will live, and the level of the available formal and informal social support.

Environmental adaptations

Minor or major adaptations to the patient's home are often required before discharge from hospital even when the residual disability is relatively mild. Learnt motor tasks, such as walking, are automatic activities and their performance normally requires minimal conscious effort by the individual. However, with impairments of perceptual and cognitive function, or even just physical or mental fatigue, more attentional effort is usually needed to perform these activities safely, despite the relatively well-preserved motor function. For example, a person with unilateral hemispatial neglect and very mild hemiparesis may trip over minor obstacles, such as a loose rug, and fall when walking unless he concentrates his attention. A pre-discharge assessment of the patient in his own home should reveal such hazards. Sometimes the provision of equipment and aids is also necessary, but care should be taken to avoid the provision of unnecessary aids and adaptations that are often powerful reminders of lost competencies and of the stigma which is sometimes associated with disability.

Support for informal carers

Informal social support in the context of healthcare is defined as the emotional, practical and informational help given to patients by their family members and friends. It is different from the interventions provided by health and social care professionals as part of their statutory duties.

Empathy, expression of concern, showing affection and giving reassurance are the main forms of emotional support. Emotional support appears to be more important than informational and practical support in the early stages of recovery from serious illness. It has been shown to reduce depressive symptoms, improve the patient's self-esteem, promote adjustment to functional loss and protect against future maladaptive behaviour, such as dependency on others. A faster and more sustained recovery is usually seen in patients who have wide social support networks, and the extent of benefit is normally proportional to the amount of support given. Interestingly, supportive behaviour is most useful when it is considered by the patients to meet their needs.

In contrast to emotional support, practical social support is most beneficial when given in moderate amounts. It is important to realise that overprotective behaviour may foster functional dependency, encourage learnt helplessness and increase reliance on others. On the other hand, inadequate practical support may lead to loss of the functional improvement that was gained before discharge from hospital.

Several reasons motivate people to become informal caregivers, including a sense of duty or loyalty and social pressure arising from other people's expectation. Carers are a valuable resource to the disabled person and to society. Their contribution should be recognised and they should be offered practical and emotional support, e.g. respite care, to reduce the stress associated with the physical demands and financial consequences of caring, and the social restrictions imposed by caring.

Follow-up after discharge from hospital
Most patients will need to attend outpatient clinics periodically after discharge from hospital. The purpose of the outpatient clinic follow-up is to monitor the patient's neurological and functional recovery, to anticipate and prevent loss of functional independence, to ensure that all the necessary lifestyles adjustments imposed by the newly acquired disability are optimal, and to prevent secondary disability, e.g. by the timely management of impairments such as severe muscle spasticity. In addition, patients frequently experience significant emotional problems

on return to their homes, mainly due to changes in their family and social roles. As these patients often require professional help to adjust better to their new disability and its social consequences, monitoring of their emotional state and coping mechanisms after discharge from hospital is an important function of the outpatient clinic. Clinic follow-up also provides the opportunity to review the adequacy of the social support to the patient and his carers that was provided at the time of hospital discharge and to provide timely interventions, if necessary.

Rehabilitation in the community

It is not necessary for patients to be in hospital until they reach their full potential of functional improvement. In fact, it is advantageous to carry out the later stages of the rehabilitation programme in the community in order to enable the patient to develop further problem-solving abilities and the use of compensatory strategies in real-life situations. Therefore, most patients will need further therapy interventions in the community. Community rehabilitation also reduces the risk of readmission to hospital by building on the functional gains acquired in hospital, and also by providing support to the patients and their carers.

The provision of emotional and practical support for patients and their carers, especially during the transition from hospital to the community, is also an important aspect of the rehabilitation programme. Many patients and their carers feel apprehensive about discharge from the safety of the hospital environment to their homes. Fear of recurrence of the disease, uncertainties about one's ability to cope at home, concerns about long-term dependency, the need to adjust to new family and social roles, and a sense of financial insecurity are common. These issues need to be addressed by the MDT. Reassurance, advice on benefits, employment, leisure activities, driving a motor vehicle and information about the community services provided by statutory and voluntary organisations are often required.

Vocational rehabilitation

Return to gainful employment is an important goal of rehabilitation, even when severe disability persists. The income from employment often secures the individual's financial independence. In addition, people in paid work usually perceive themselves as valued members of society. This fosters a belief of self-worth and often enhances self-esteem. Other possible benefits of employment include the opportunity for social contacts and meaningful, structured time occupation. Long-term unemployment frequently results in financial dependency (on the State or on family members) and is associated with low mood and poor self-esteem. All of these factors may lead to social isolation. Disabled patients who are not of retirement age should therefore be encouraged to return to work.

The initial assessment for return to work is usually started in the hospital's occupational therapy department. This should preferably be followed by a direct observation of the patient's performance in the workplace. Liaison at an early stage with the occupational health team of the patient's employers is essential. The aim of this assessment is to establish the patient's ability to attend for work reliably, his behaviour in the workplace (including his interaction with work colleagues and customers), his productivity, the impact of fatigue on his performance, and the need for supervision or practical support. The assessment should also include whether adaptations to the work environment would be necessary. In addition to the information derived from this assessment, the employer should also be advised on whether the patient has any residual disability, its nature and prognosis, and the need for ongoing therapy. In complex cases, the advice of a qualified and experienced occupational health physician may be necessary.

When vocational rehabilitation is required, it is best delivered through an employer-based programme, whenever possible. In some cases, graded return to work may be necessary. Some patients may be able to do only flexible hours, part-time work or work from home; this needs to be negotiated with employers either directly or through a statutory organisation, such as the Disability Advisory Service.

Supported employment and sheltered employment schemes (i.e. work in non-industrial settings) may be considered if the patient is not able to carry out his previous job, or an alternative perhaps less demanding work in the competitive market.

Leisure activities

Hobbies and other leisure pursuits are pleasurable activities to the individual. They alleviate boredom and enable people to use their spare time in a way that is meaningful to them. Furthermore, they often provide opportunities for socialisation and friendships. Some leisure pursuits, especially outdoor activities, may also have additional health benefits. An important goal of rehabilitation is to help patients occupy their spare time and enable them to pursue their previous hobbies and leisure activities, or to develop new ones. Numerous voluntary organisations in the UK provide leisure facilities and organise leisure activities for people with disabilities of all ages.

The role of social services and voluntary organisations

People with disabilities are often socially isolated. Many factors may contribute to this, including the loss of physical independence, depression, poor motivation, low self-esteem and financial difficulties. In the UK, social services departments of Local Authorities and many voluntary organisations offer services for disabled individuals and to their carers in 'Day Centres', 'Stroke Clubs', etc., and in supported employment schemes. These services provide emotional and practical support to patients and their families and, in addition, they help to reduce their social isolation.

INDEX